OLDER YET FASTER

*The Secret to Running Fast
and Injury Free*

Second edition

Keith Bateman and Heidi Jones

© Keith Bateman and Heidi Jones 2018
© Illustrations, Ainsley Knott 2018
Older Yet Faster Publications Pty Ltd
olderyetfaster.com

All rights reserved. Except for short passages for reviews, no part of this publication in any of its formats may be used in any way without written permission of the publisher.

First published in Australia in 2014
Second edition published in Australia 2018

ISBN: 978-0-9941921-8-9

Dewey number: 796.42071
Editing: Jamie Roberts and Rubida Communications
Illustrations: Ainsley Knott
Cover design: Stuart Greaves
Book internal design and production management: Rubida Communications

Disclaimer
Running is a personal journey for which you must take responsibility. This book cannot take into account your individual physical or medical situation. Check with your medical professional before starting or amending any exercise program. The publisher and the authors accept no liability for loss or injury resulting from using the contents of this book.

ACKNOWLEDGEMENTS

Many people have helped us in many ways with both the first edition and this second edition.

Thanks to Mick Chay, Alison Mead, Martin Cosby, Melanie Barton, Andrew Halliday, Paul Simpson, Robert Miller and Keith's son, James Bateman, for help with the first edition. And for the second edition, thanks to Tony Guttmann and Mark Conyers for their detailed analysis of our drafts, Lena Fleming for suggesting and helping with the new cover design, and David Blackman for blogging his technique-change experiences following the first edition.

Ainsley (ainsleyknott.com), you have brought this book alive with your excellent illustrations. You accurately interpreted our ideas and responded to our changing needs with grace and professionalism.

Our thanks also goes to Stuart Greaves for allowing us to use his pictures of Keith and Heidi on the front and back covers, and to Steven and Lena at Xero Shoes for the footwear.

An extra special thank you must go to our friend and mentor Robert Miller, who has dedicated more than three years to brilliantly drawing out our passion for what we do, and assisting us to express ourselves more clearly. You have helped ensure that this second edition is more detailed, comprehensive and has a more personal touch. Spending hours with you deliberating over sometimes only a few sentences was great fun and highly rewarding.

From Keith

Thanks also goes to my coach, Sean Williams, who for over 15 years has guided, pushed, and restrained me. Sean, I really appreciate your wisdom. It has been an honour to run with Sean's Elite squad since 2003, which included some of Australia's best runners, such as

Australian 10,000 metre record holder Ben St Lawrence, Harry Summers and Neil Berry.

Apart from running with, chasing and being chased by these runners, including Sean himself, it has been a buzz to have a wonderful string of 'training buddies' to train and race with over the years. These included Belinda (Belzy) Wilsher, twice City2Surf (Sydney) winner Lara Tamsett, Jim (Bruiser) Dawes, Tom Hurley, Morgan MacDonald, Martin Matthews, Mick Chay, Rob Lansdown, Tony (Fats) Fattorini, and many, many more. Also, watching and mentoring the youngsters in the squad and being their 'target' in training until they were fast enough to pass me has been like being a dad again.

Eloise Wellings, thanks for the privilege of being your training partner in the weeks before the 2012 Olympics, and Liz Miller, Clare Geraghty, Lara Tamsett and Becky Lowe, thanks for letting me pace you in the City2Surf and other races. It's been a ball and long may it continue—I intend to be running with you guys for many more years—so watch your backs, your conscience isn't far behind!

James and Andy Polson, without you I would never have started on this project. It was you who first approached me with the idea of producing an iPhone app. You helped a great deal with the structure of the first edition.

And to my best friend and now my wife, Heidi Jones, many thanks for your expert podiatry advice, enthusiasm, brilliant steering of this project, and for keeping the pressure on and working with me to finish this book.

From Heidi

My deepest thanks go to my soul mate Keith. Not only have you helped many of my patients, you have also resuscitated my running life. After so many injuries, I lost belief in myself as an athlete. I thought I couldn't change my technique. I have learnt so much from you, and you have transformed the way I assess and treat my running patients. Through technique change everyone can run smoother, faster and avoid unnecessary injuries.

A big thank you to the gurus in their fields: Pilates teacher Gataneo del Monaco for guiding me towards starting a foot strengthening program;

Angelo Castiglione for his self-myofascial release therapy advice; running coach Alan McCloskey for his foot exercises; and osteopath and runner Dr Chris Jones, not only for his rehabilitation exercises but also for the many times he has put my broken body back together. My journey has led me to these great people and you will find their exercises in *Heidi's Strengthening Program* and *Heidi's rehabilitation exercises*.

And finally, a big thank you to my father who made me fall in love with running from a very young age. You guided and nurtured my competitive spirit, which not only led me to achieve good results in running but has also helped me during the difficult times in life. Thanks dad!

TESTIMONIALS

Based on the first edition

> 'Older Yet Faster sets the new standard for running technique training and theory. Whilst tackling the most essential tenet of our sport, this book can teach any level of runner or coach the correct technique to run quickly and efficiently. Keith and Heidi, with their years of record-breaking running, show the reader how to become faster and remain injury free. This book has been an amazing help to me as a coach, and to countless runners whom I coach. I recommend this book as a helpful guide on running technique and to anyone who wants to get faster by following some simple measures.'

Sean Williams has been a regular Australian Athletics Team coach at the World Athletics Championships, World Cross-country Championships and International Ekiden relays. Sean has coached three Commonwealth Games athletes, with two also being Olympians. Sean has been Keith and Heidi's coach for many years.

> 'I can wholeheartedly recommend Older Yet Faster. As a long-time ultramarathon runner, I had picked up some bad habits, leading me to an inefficient running style and ultimately to injuries. By following the drills and techniques in Older Yet Faster, I have experienced a transformation in my running and a heightened awareness of body balance whilst running. The transformation from rhino to gazelle takes commitment and patience, but check out Keith's running style and I guarantee you will think "I want to run like that!"'

Lisa Harvey-Smith, MPhys (Hons), PhD, astrophysicist, ultramarathon runner and author. Lisa has completed a gruelling 250 kilometre race through Australia's Simpson desert and several 100-kilometre, 6-hour, 12-hour and 24-hour races. She is a member of the Australian Ultra-runners Association's '100 club' for athletes who have completed 100 miles in under 24 hours.

> 'What have you got to lose by buying this book? For me, it was 20 seconds off my 4:30 endurance pace simply by adopting its simple technique change. This change also helped me run 2:48:36 at the 2015 Gold Coast Marathon; a massive 19 minute personal best and number 7 world ranking for my age-group. Considering I am 62 (older than Keith) and have only been a runner for less than 3 years, you can definitely take my word for it that it will be money well spent.'

John Shaw, Brisbane, Queensland, Australia

> 'Absolutely Fantastic Book. Profoundly simple in theory and application. With my professional background in sports rehabilitation and a long association with distance running, I will be recommending this book to all of my clients as "The Must Read Book on Running" in 2015.'

Ian Fischer, Adv. Dip. RM (Myotherapy), Central West Myotherapy, Orange, New South Wales, Australia

> 'I received your ebook yesterday, had a quick flick through, went for my usual 5.8 kilometre time trial tonight. I tried to remember what I'd read and put some of it into practice, lost it quite a lot but felt right part of the time. Took 49 seconds off previous personal best. I'm in my late 70s and haven't improved for a long time—very happy. Now to read it more thoroughly!'

Sheila, Western Australia

> 'Of all the running books, this is one I come back to again and again (usually before a race!). The principles are beautifully explained and easy to understand. The first week I worked with Keith, I took 90 seconds off my 10 kilometre time. Since then I've taken another 2 minutes off. I've sliced 30 minutes off my marathon time, to run in the low 2:40s. Running great has three

elements: get an awesome coach, get your form efficient and have fun. With this book you'll be on your way.'

Rhett Gibson, age 32, Sydney, New South Wales, Australia

TABLE OF CONTENTS

Acknowledgements iii
    From Keith iii
    From Heidi iv
Testimonials vi
    Based on the first edition vi
Foreword xiii
About the authors xvii
    Keith Bateman, competitor and coach xvii
    Heidi Jones, rehabilitation specialist and podiatrist xx
About this book xxv
    Second edition xxv
    Who is this book for? xxv
    How to use this book xxvi
Chapter 1 How poor technique affects your running 1
    1.1 Poor technique is mainly due to over-striding 2
    1.2 How to check if you are over-striding 5
    1.3 Recognising the signs of poor technique 6
    1.4 Run, don't walk 12
Chapter 2 Poor technique causes injuries 15
    2.1 Injuries to the feet 16
    2.2 Injuries to the rest of the body 19
    2.3 Dealing with injuries 24

Chapter 3 Good technique—how it works 27
   3.1 Landing 28
   3.2 Take-off 32
   3.3 Accelerating 37
Chapter 4 Introducing Keith's Lessons 39
Chapter 5 Lesson One: Landing 43
Chapter 6 Lesson Two: Take-off 49
   6.1 Before you start 49
   6.2 Using the bounce 50
   6.3 Moving off in good form 52
   6.4 Single-leg start 52
   6.5 Summary 54
Chapter 7 Lesson Three: Accelerating 55
   7.1 Accelerating by taking off more strongly 55
   7.2 Accelerating by tilting more 57
   7.3 Accelerating by raising the back foot 59
   7.4 Summary 60
Chapter 8 Lesson Four: Keith's Game Changer 61
   8.1 Preparation 61
   8.2 Finding your balance point 63
   8.3 Summary 65
Chapter 9 Lesson Five: Going for a run 67
   9.1 Checking your form 68
   9.2 What should happen during your run 70
   9.3 Running hills 73
   9.4 Summary 76

Chapter 10 Lesson Six: Maintaining good form 77
   10.1 Ways to check your form during your run *77*
   10.2 Other checks and exercises to refine your form *84*
   10.3 Summary *90*

Chapter 11 Heidi's Strengthening Program 91
   11.1 Strengthening your feet *92*
   11.2 Strengthening your glutes *104*

Chapter 12 Managing your transition 107
   12.1 Changes to expect *107*
   12.2 The stages of the transition *108*
   12.3 Main points to look out for in your transition *110*

Chapter 13 Heidi's rehabilitation exercises 113
   13.1 Transitional soreness *114*
   13.2 More serious injuries *115*

Chapter 14 Shoes—what you need to know 125
   14.1 'Technology' in shoes is never beneficial *126*
   14.2 Our guide to shoes *127*
   14.3 Orthotics *136*

Chapter 15 How to get a hot runner's body 139
   15.1 Body strength through running *140*
   15.2 Things you don't need to worry about *140*
   15.3 How do you spot a good runner? *142*

Chapter 16 Tips and traps 147
   16.1 General training tips *147*
   16.2 'I am different', 'I can't run because ...'. *148*
   16.3 Care for your body *149*
   16.4 Racing *150*
   16.5 Trails *151*

16.6 Don't neglect side-view video reviews *151*

16.7 Don't force changes to your cadence *152*

16.8 Don't sweat about your 'vertical oscillation' *154*

16.9 Don't change your foot strike *154*

16.10 Don't try to 'fall forwards' *154*

16.11 Don't just copy others *155*

16.12 Don't be conned into setting the wrong goals *155*

16.13 Don't be swayed by sales gimmicks *156*

16.14 Where you might go wrong *157*

Appendix A For coaches—applying the lessons 158

Appendix B For podiatrists—treating runners 171

Appendix C Heidi's Strengthening Program explained 189

Appendix D Summary of OYF Rules 197

Appendix E Kilometres to miles conversion chart 202

Commonly used terms 203

References 206

List of illustrations 207

List of exercises 213

Index 215

FOREWORD

Stuart Greaves

This book is for everyone who runs, or wants to run, as they did as a child at home in the back yard—carefree and quite possibly barefoot too. I have rediscovered the joy of running barefoot at the local oval, just as we all did as little kids.

The principles that Keith and Heidi describe apply to all runners, from overweight reformed-smoker back-of-the-packers to would-be Olympians. Heidi and Keith are passionate about their craft. That is why they take care to accommodate runners from whatever level they are coming from.

Everyone needs to progress at their own pace and obviously that will vary enormously between individuals. The overweight will need to be especially cautious as the loads on their frame and joints will be greater, the strains on their less-developed muscles, ligaments and tendons will manifest earlier, and they will have to make the transition in a very careful, gradual way. Even elite runners will need to be careful with any changes they make, as they already have high power and endurance, and any change can possibly be reflected in increased loading on some other part of the body. Change starts immediately, but you must be patient. Too much enthusiasm, too much too soon, can cause injury. I regularly receive scoldings from Heidi for overdoing it. You have been warned. Don't annoy her.

It also won't take long before you notice Keith and Heidi spend a lot of time barefoot, or in the lightest, flattest shoes you can imagine. It is surprising to see Keith advocating running barefoot on not just grass and soft surfaces, but on concrete as well. And yet, when you examine his feet, his soles are not hard, calloused or blistered. But let's be sensible, in the backyard at home the worst that can happen barefoot is treading on some sharp bits of the kids' Lego. On the streets, obviously the hazards are real—gravel, glass, the ubiquitous McDonalds detritus, doggie dos. Yuck! So you will need shoes as well.

I also don't believe this style of 'natural' running is just the latest fad in a fashion and sales-driven industry. Discussing elements of this book with medical professionals has sometimes evoked a reaction along the lines of: 'If you try to run barefoot or in those ridiculous finger shoes, all I can say is I'll have plenty of business from you.' The suggestion is that the kind of running described in this book will cause injury, rather than prevent it. Most often, the people who make such remarks, even though they might be highly credentialed physicians, are not serious runners. But in one aspect they are correct. Too much change too soon and you will be sitting on the couch nursing a new niggling injury, most likely a strained calf muscle or a sore Achilles tendon. But, if you follow the principles in Keith's Lessons and use Heidi's Strengthening Program, then there is no reason why your running cannot be injury free.

Advertising says to wear soft, comfortable shoes with lots of support to 'control' your feet. Like Keith and Heidi, I have come to believe the opposite is true. I spent many years carrying running injuries that I now believe were preventable. The rigid orthotics I used for years temporarily addressed one problem, but created a lot more. And when I threw them away and strengthened weak muscles rather than pandering to a specific weakness, I started my transition to real speed.

Keith and Heidi write about their area of expertise: running performance and injury prevention. This book doesn't give lengthy connect-the-dots training schedules. While the principles apply to all, there can't be a one-size-fits-all program for your training schedule. Neither does this book give you a program to give up smoking or drinking, or to help you revise your nutrition or lose weight, important though they are.

While you may want to improve your breathing and overall health by taking up a no-smoking program, you can still eat, drink and be merry. Regarding dieting, I'd suggest you don't need to worry too much about your weight. Once you start training sensibly and consistently, if you eat good food in moderation and resist any binge eating or drinking, the weight falls off naturally.

I wasn't a schoolboy athlete. I only started running in my twenties. When I moved to long distances in 1980, I spent a few years trying to break three hours for the marathon, which is a pretty decent goal for any runner. But this goal eluded me no matter how hard I flogged myself with all those long slow distance miles. Running 3:00:42 in the Big-M Melbourne marathon was particularly annoying. All I wanted back then was to improve by just one lousy minute. Roll forwards eight years and by the time I turned 30, with a change in technique and approach, I had broken three hours not just by a few seconds, but by well over half an hour.

To what do I attribute this substantial improvement? Three things. Firstly, very gradually changing my technique. This really helped prevent injury, as I learnt to adapt to all those hours of training. Secondly, placing greater emphasis on running fast with the greatest possible efficiency. It's not about just more and more mileage. It's about technique. And that's where this book will give you a huge head-start. The third element was spending as much time as possible with better runners and just trying to keep up. Watch, learn, compete, repeat. Now, at the age of 60, I am re-inspired by Keith's amazing world record age-group performances. With this book, I now have another important tool in keeping injury at bay and getting fast again. I hope you also will be inspired.

There's one more thing. Observing Keith and Heidi in training, I have been surprised at how much can be achieved with relatively little distance. Decades ago, we all used to believe that you had to flog yourself with big mileages each week to be a fast distance runner. It struck me recently that once the technique is spot on, good results can be achieved with not a lot of mileage. It's amazing how fast these two are, even when running as little as 15 or 20 kilometres per week. Sometimes, after warm-up, exercises and a few drills, we'll ease through just a dozen barefoot laps of the oval before heading to a local cafe. Maybe four or five kilometres. That's been quite a revelation. Years ago, I know they also spent decades running well over 100 kilometres per week, but it's quite refreshing to realise that we can still run, and race, pretty fast without having to grind out all that distance stuff. So in reading this book, you won't find regimented training programs that tell you exactly how much time or distance to spend in training. It seems that is very much an individual thing. But once the technique is spot on, less is indeed more. It's time for a cappuccino!

Stuart Greaves
49 marathons completed, 2:22 marathon (1987)

ABOUT THE AUTHORS

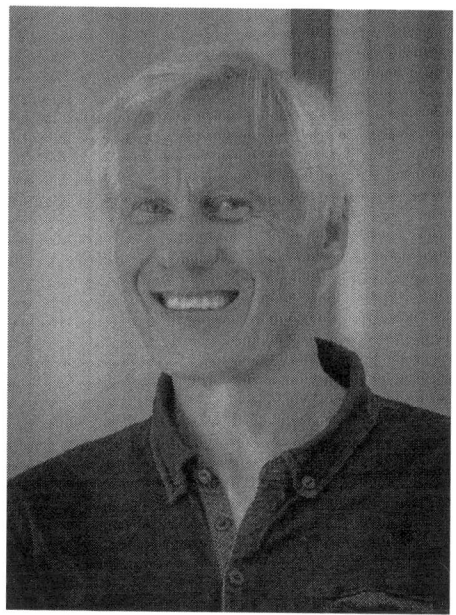

Keith Bateman. Photo by Stuart Greaves.

Keith Bateman, competitor and coach

I was born in Watford and I became interested in skiing on the artificial slopes around London.

I qualified as a ski instructor and moved up to Scotland to teach downhill skiing in 1979. My interest in running started five years later when I entered a local fun run to get into shape for cross-country ski racing the following winter. I did quite well and with a rush of enthusiasm I entered the Glasgow Marathon. The irony is, I now advise people to make sure to build up towards longer races over many years, in order to avoid injuries.

On the entry form, I predicted my time to be around 3:15 based on my training times and so I started well back in the large field. I was delighted to pass people all the way and to finish well ahead of my expectations in 2:49. It was obviously faster to run with others on tarmac than alone in the forests and glens of the Scottish Highlands. A month later, I ran the tough Black Isle Marathon near Inverness, finishing in a good time of 2:44. Now running was in my blood, but I wasn't as obsessed with running as I am now.

The next step was to join a club, which happened to be Inverness Harriers. I started running in races over different distances and terrain, including the Highland Cross and other mountain races, and even a few triathlons. I ran over 5 kilometres, 10 kilometres (36:36 on the road was my best time) and half-marathons, and from 1996 onwards I was very active on the Scottish Hill Race scene. However, despite my interest in running, I pushed it into the background for long periods of time due to my very busy lifestyle. At this stage of my life, I was renovating houses, raising a family, operating a ski school and running a sports hire shop. Without giving myself time to train properly, I gained 15 kilograms in weight and my fitness dropped significantly.

In 2000, I emigrated to Australia at the age of 45 and I got back into running by joining Sydney Striders running club. I felt very uneasy being out of condition, so I was highly motivated to regain my peak fitness. I didn't realise how far I had to go until I entered a 10-kilometre race, only to find that I struggled; my time was a very slow 43:32—there was serious work to be done!

I continued to run with my club and, although I did improve a fair bit, I knew I could run faster. I also knew I couldn't do that without getting some outside help, so I began to look around for a coach. I got lucky. I was introduced to Sean Williams and started training with his squad in October 2003. This was a prestigious group, which contained several future Olympians. I was determined to make the most of the opportunity to learn all I could from these elite runners and so I paid close attention to how they were running. I may have overdone it, as with the increased training load I started to pick up injuries. I was a classic heel-striker without knowing it and my running was frequently interrupted with knee, iliotibial band, hip flexor and shin pain. I was able to keep running with short lay-offs, but my main frustration was that I was unable to get faster. I gradually incorporated small changes into my own technique and, although my times continued to improve, these improvements were only modest.

In 2007, I went off to get a biomechanical assessment and received a detailed report and a set of strengthening exercises. I tried to adhere to them, but my running times were no better. However, this last-ditch attempt to improve my speed did yield a result. It made me realise that if I was going to succeed, I needed to concentrate on the efficiency of my running action rather than trying to build up strength. My eureka moment came when I realised that the simple root cause preventing me and other runners from achieving more was not weakness but poor technique. It was commonly believed that it was lack of strength that held runners back and resulted in injuries. I realised it was poor technique that not only leads to slower times, but also causes the stress that leads to injury. I got stronger and fixed my injuries simply by fixing my technique.

I had set a few New South Wales state records from May 2004, but it was when the technique changes came that I started knocking minutes off those times. The records that I set in the 55-age-group were faster than the existing records in the 45-age-group. At the time of writing, I have broken, and still hold, 38 age-group New South Wales state records, 15 Australian age-group records and five 55-age-group world records: 1500 metres (4:12:35), 1 mile (4:35:04), 3000 metres (8:56:80), 5000 metres (15:29:7) and 10,000 metres (31:51:86).

Now that I had worked out how to run with good technique, it was only a matter of time and small adjustments until I developed my own my technique-change lessons. I stayed with Sean's group and, in 2011, Sean suggested that I start some of my own coaching sessions to relieve him of some of his workload.

Finally, I got lucky yet again when I met Heidi. Among other things, she had developed her strengthening and rehabilitation exercises, which fitted in and completed my running system. I formalised my knowledge of good technique and the correct way of running in 2014 when I published the first edition of this book with my wife Heidi. Heidi's Strengthening Program rounds out a complete guide to transitioning into good form, and Heidi's rehabilitation exercises help with transition, and with rehabilitation from injury.

I currently conduct private coaching sessions and teach running at a Sydney secondary school, where I help my runners by changing their technique and getting them into low-profile shoes. I am excited that my lessons combine so well with Heidi's Strengthening Program to provide runners with a comprehensive system that can help them run smoother and faster and, hopefully, injury free.

Heidi Jones, rehabilitation specialist and podiatrist

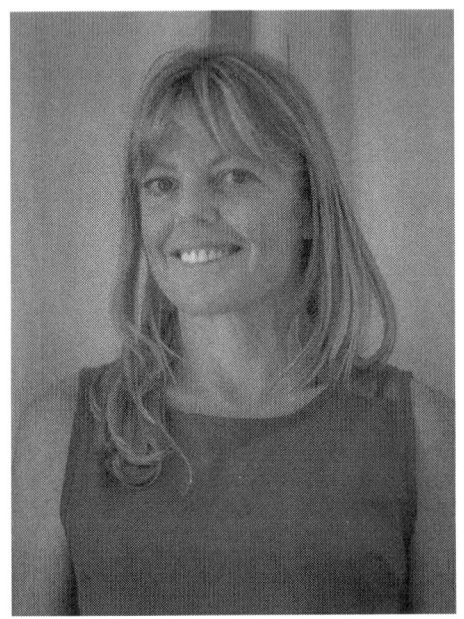

Heidi Jones (Dip. Pod., MA Pod. A). Photo by Stuart Greaves.

I developed a passion for running at a very early age. My father was a physical education teacher and, as a family, we all participated in a wide range of sports. I found that running came easily to me. With the running boom in the 1980s, our family ended up travelling all over the state to compete in fun runs every couple of weekends. Before long, I was keeping up with the big boys and, what started off as spending time with my dad, developed into a high level of achievement by the age of 17.

In 1991, I achieved a number of notable results. In that year, I won many races in both under-20s and open competitions. I was Combined Schools State Champion over 3000 metres on the track, and All Schools

State Champion over 4 kilometres in the cross-country. I even came third in the Australian Cross-country Championships (under-20s), but I was also performing well over longer distances and my times were extremely competitive. For example, I won the Parramatta Open in a record time of 58:13 for 10 miles and set a very fast time and personal best of 33:40 for 10 kilometres in a Sydney road race. As a result of these achievements, I was awarded the 1991 New South Wales Open Female Runner of the Year.

However, towards the end of that year, tragedy struck. I got out of bed one morning and I couldn't put any weight on my left forefoot. It was very painful and swollen and incredibly tender to touch. I was repeatedly misdiagnosed by various doctors. Apparently, I was suffering from gout, arthritis, a stress fracture, or it was just 'bruising'. I was even told it was psychosomatic (I was making it up!). It was an incredibly traumatic time for a girl who just wanted to run.

It took 12 months before I was correctly diagnosed as having a genetic bone disorder in the ball of my foot (Freiberg's disease). I was then told by three orthopaedic surgeons that I would never run again, and that there was no operation for it. However, I managed to finally find the one and only surgeon in the Southern Hemisphere who could fix this, Dr Kim Slater. I was delighted that his surgery allowed me to walk again, but what I desperately wanted to do was to run.

For the first year or so, I was prescribed an orthotic with a metatarsal dome to take the pressure off the second toe area. This was very successful and I started walking long distances to get back into condition and, after three long years, at the age of 21, I could finally resume running.

I continued to use orthotics for several years but, after sustaining seven tibial stress fractures in a row, I threw them out in exasperation. Amazingly, the stress fractures stopped. This experience led me to question whether the orthotics really were the answer to fast, injury-free running. Definitely not in my case. Something wasn't adding up and I wanted to find out why.

I decided to train as a podiatrist—in Australia, a podiatrist diagnoses, treats and prevents injuries to the feet and lower limbs—and learn how to treat injuries so that other teenagers didn't have to go through what I went through. I started my own clinic in 2000 and continued to work my way up to senior podiatrist at St Vincent's Hospital's high-risk foot clinic in Sydney. I was there for 19 years until 2016.

Meanwhile, I was still running in thick chunky shoes 'for support', and although I didn't sustain any more stress fractures, I continued to suffer many injuries from over-striding (landing with the foot too far in front of the hips). For example, iliotibial band friction syndrome (which plagued me for years), bursitis of the hip (nine months off), and runner's knee (eight months off). I was determined to find a way out of this nightmare. I took myself off to yoga, Pilates and the gym to strengthen my body and core stability, and to improve my posture. I also found that roller therapy (self-myofascial release therapy), which 'irons out' the fascia, was great for smoothing out tight iliotibial bands. Unfortunately, although these things were very beneficial, much of the time I was treating my symptoms and getting short-term relief without addressing the cause.

My future looked bleak. I was in a world of pain and, if I continued down this track, I would have done irreparable damage and sunk further into depression. I just couldn't get off the ground. Fortunately, my luck changed in one of those chance meetings that transforms your life. I joined Sean Williams' running group and I met Keith Bateman. Watching him run, and eventually learning his methods, would lead to my salvation.

Keith was lapping me in training and it didn't sit well. I used to race men as a teenager; it was such fun beating them, but I knew I would never beat this one. He trained barefoot on the grass and in the thinnest shoes on the road. I marvelled at how a (then) 55-year-old man kept getting faster and faster! He wasn't just a good club runner, he was blowing my own personal best times out of the water!

I had to find out what his secret was, and so I enrolled in one of his group technique sessions. At the outset he suggested we remove our shoes and do the session barefoot. He took us through a series of very specific drills, which seemed easy at the time, but for the next two weeks the muscles in my feet and my calves were so sore I could hardly walk. I wasn't too sure about this barefoot running and I decided to have a one-on-one session with him.

Keith filmed me from the side and I asked him why. He smiled and said, 'I wanted to see where your foot lands in relation to your hips.' He drew a line through my image and I could see my foot was landing way in front of my hips. This simple observation was very powerful. As podiatrists, in our biomechanics classes, we were taught to view and assess the patient from the front/back (anterior/posterior) view. There was no mention in my studies about the foot needing to land under the hips. Equally important, there was no mention of how damaging over-striding really is.

We were taught to control excessive pronation (the foot rolling inward towards the inner edge of the sole) and other ailments by placing a hard thermoplastic device, known as an orthotic, in the running shoe. However, Keith's approach is radically different. It is so simple yet so effective. It gets to the core of most runners' problems. He is treating the cause of almost all running-related injuries. He teaches that by landing with your foot under your hips, you reduce excessive pronation and the multitude of injuries related to excessive pronation. Most of the measurements taken in biomechanical assessments then become irrelevant.

Using the running technique that I was taught in podiatry school, it was always a mystery to me why I got injured. However, I can now see that my massive over-stride meant I was hitting the ground hard. As my fitness improved, I went faster and so I hit the ground even harder causing my body to break down. Not being able to walk properly for two weeks after just one barefoot session shocked me into realising how weak my calf and feet muscles were. I had been running for 30 years! How could this be? I blame my weak feet on supportive running shoes and orthotics, which I wore from my mid-teens. At last a lifelong mystery was solved.

All my adult running life I have been told I over-pronated and I needed support. The irony is, wearing thick chunky supportive shoes actually made me pronate even more. Raising the heel of the shoe forced my foot to hit the ground early, with a force equivalent to several times my body weight. My whole body was pushed out of alignment: I was bent at the waist, and this in turn caused me to hunch my shoulders. I had tight neck muscles for 25 years. We show how this happens later in the book.

Originally, I thought that I could find a solution to my injury problems by studying podiatry, but it was only now that I was in a position to do this. With the insights that I gained from Keith, combined with the knowledge I gained from trying to deal with my own injuries, I knew what I needed to do. I went right back to basics. It was time to strengthen my feet and to take a more holistic approach. I was guided by my Pilates instructor to develop a foot strengthening program.

I tried it out myself and, not only did my feet feel amazing, I could also see the arches in my feet developing nicely. I started offering this as an alternative to orthotics and received amazing feedback. No runner has opted for orthotics since. I work closely with Keith, stressing the importance of technique-change sessions, and I am up-front with my patients, telling them that they must drastically cut down mileage while their feet and calf muscles adapt. Footwear is also important, especially the shoes that are worn during the day. I get my patients into thin, flat, flexible shoes with no heel, so that their spine is vertical and their postural muscles are engaged. I wear thin, flat, flexible shoes to work. Since wearing a thinner shoe, together with technique change, I have not experienced knee, iliotibial band, hip or back pain.

I did have some pain and stiffness in my calf muscles and foot arches while I adapted, but I carefully managed this and now I feel strong and confident. My running is fluid and I am finding it difficult to run slowly! For the first time in my life, I am not worried about getting injured. I went from 4:10 per kilometre down to 3:40 for my 1-kilometre repetitions within a few weeks. I had found the 'sweet spot' by landing balanced.

However, my return to competitive running has been delayed. In February 2014, I became seriously ill from life-threatening food poisoning. It went into my blood and left me with bacterial-induced chronic fatigue. To this day, I cannot work a full day. I have also had to tailor my training around my energy levels. It has taken me four years to be able to run three times a week and only in short quality sessions, but I am slowly recovering and am now able to run four times per week.

As well as fixing foot problems, I am also a devoted runner and my experience in podiatry puts me in the perfect position to help my running patients by teaching them my unique foot strengthening exercises. I also help them to transition away from orthotics and get them into thin, flat, flexible shoes for normal use as well as for running. It is gratifying that everyone has responded extremely well to my Spiky Ball and Foot Program exercises, and so far no-one has ever asked to continue wearing orthotics.

ABOUT THIS BOOK

Keith Bateman and Heidi Jones

Second edition

We are absolutely delighted with the response to the first edition and the results it has produced for our readers. It is very encouraging that physicists and engineers are at the forefront of the excellent feedback. However, in line with our desire for perfection, this second edition incorporates some amendments.

We have noted readers' comments and experiences, and refined the text and illustrations accordingly. In some emails, readers have said things that indicate they might have misinterpreted something, or they have used terminology which we feel they might have misunderstood. Also, Keith continues to improve his technique sessions. Some of the changes made in this second edition reflect these refinements. He has also added a section specifically for coaches who want to teach OYF Running.

We have introduced some new illustrations to expand our ideas in certain areas, mostly concerning shoes and how they affect your posture. Heidi has refined her strengthening program, added a chapter on rehabilitation and written a chapter for podiatrists.

We hope you enjoy our work!

Who is this book for?

Older Yet Faster (OYF) is a manual for teaching runners how to transition to efficient running using the OYF Running technique and help them avoid incurring almost all of the common running injuries as they do so. The book is ideal for beginners to learn how to run well, and for experienced runners to change over to good technique. Coaches can also use this book as a reference on how to implement technique change for their clients, and we expect it will become the go-to manual for medical and allied health professionals to help them deal with running-related injuries caused by bad technique and poor footwear choices.

You will bring with you your own running experience, either from reading articles, talking with friends or from your own training. If you are changing your technique, it is important that you follow Keith's Lessons carefully, as any preconceived ideas can be easily mixed up with the true message. To remove any confusion, we have included our 'OYF Rules' throughout the chapters. These rules emphasise the important aspects of what we are teaching. We list them again at the back of the book in Appendix D, so you can reference them in one place.

How to use this book

Before starting the exercises, we thoroughly recommend that everyone reads the first three chapters, which analyse the elements of running technique and the importance of overcoming the main problem of over-striding. After gaining a good understanding of running technique, you will be prepared to read about our technique-change system, which we call OYF Running. This consists of Keith's Lessons used in combination with Heidi's Strengthening Program and forms the main body of the book.

Chapter 4 is a short introduction to Keith's Lessons, which are a set of six lessons presented in chapters 5 to 10 using a step-by-step guide to running with good technique. Each lesson provides exercises set out in a format that is both easy to understand and implement. The first three lessons teach you the basics of running correctly and the last three help you put these into practice and help you to refine your technique over the period of your transition. The techniques learnt in the early lessons are incorporated in the later lessons, and so the chapters and exercises should be done in sequence. After you have been through all the lessons once, you can practice any exercise in any order. Keith's Lessons are set up so that runners can teach themselves in conjunction with the online videos and forum, which are accessible from our website, olderyetfaster.com.

Heidi's Strengthening Program (Chapter 11) consists of a well-ordered series of exercises, which will help your body safely adjust to the redistribution of the workload and are essential to rebuild parts of the body which have been neglected due to poor technique. You should start Heidi's Strengthening Program as soon as possible, preferably *before* starting Keith's Lessons, in order to build strength and to deal with the resultant muscle and tendon soreness that you will start to experience.

In Chapter 2 and throughout other chapters in the book, we identify specific injuries and how they are caused, and we show how—by improving running technique and re-strengthening—these injuries are quickly cured. Podiatrists will find Heidi's experiences and advice particularly interesting, especially as these will almost certainly be in conflict with what is still taught in universities.

Chapter 12, *Managing your transition*, and Chapter 13, *Heidi's rehabilitation exercises*, explain what should happen during the transition and what to do should you get injured, or if you are currently injured. Chapter 14, *Shoes—what you need to know*, is very important, as you must have suitable footwear to run with good technique.

There is then a chapter (Chapter 15, *How to get a hot runner's body*) on how your body shape will change as you adopt your new technique, and a chapter (Chapter 16, *Tips and traps*) on general tips and traps that runners fall into.

Finally, we have included appendices for coaches, for podiatrists and a detailed look at Heidi's Strengthening Program. In Appendix A, Keith discusses how to implement Keith's Lessons from a coach's point of view; in Appendix B, Heidi explains how she treats her patients who are suffering with specific injuries; and in Appendix C, she explains Heidi's Strengthening Program in greater detail for medical professionals and interested runners. For readers who are more familiar with miles, we have also provided a conversion chart from kilometres to miles in Appendix E.

At the back of the book, there is a list of commonly used terms, a reference list, lists of illustrations and exercises, and an index.

CHAPTER 1 HOW POOR TECHNIQUE AFFECTS YOUR RUNNING

Keith Bateman and Heidi Jones

If you are new to running, you most probably will not have built strength in the right places, nor will you have acquired the knowledge of how to run correctly, and so this chapter will be relevant to you as well as more experienced runners. There is no need to head off to the gym to build up your core strength. This will come over time, from your running. What is essential is that you start with the correct running action or what we term 'good technique'. Indeed, if you have picked up this book as a new runner you have the distinct advantage of not having to un-learn bad habits.

If you have been running for a while, you might feel that you are running quite well at the moment, and you may be satisfied with your times, but if you are running with poor technique then you are not only holding yourself back but you are significantly increasing your risk of injury.

If you experience any of the effects of poor technique that we list in the next chapter, then you are facing the same problem that all runners encounter at some stage: over-striding. This action causes too much braking, excess energy use and leads to most running-related injuries; and, importantly, fixing over-striding goes a long way to correcting other errors in your running technique. Changing your running technique should also prevent you from incurring any of the injuries that we detail in the next chapter.

In this chapter, we start by analysing the three types of over-stride. We then look at signs of poor technique and encourage you to start looking at your own running action, so that you can recognise any problems that you may have. This is the first necessary step before you can learn good technique through the lessons. Finally, we look at the differences between actions of walking and running, as another way of helping you recognise and correct errors in your running technique. Throughout the chapter, we also introduce you to the first five of the ten Older Yet Faster Rules (OYF Rules). The full set of rules is given at the back of the book in Appendix D.

1.1 Poor technique is mainly due to over-striding

Over-striding is the common situation where a runner's foot is making firm contact with the ground too far in front of the runner's hips.

As can be seen in *Illustration 1*, there are three basic types of over-stride: heel (left figure), midfoot (middle figure) and forefoot (right figure). Heel and forefoot are the most common and the most damaging, but some runners have a midfoot over-stride. In each case, the runner is leaning back as they land. This causes them to slow down.

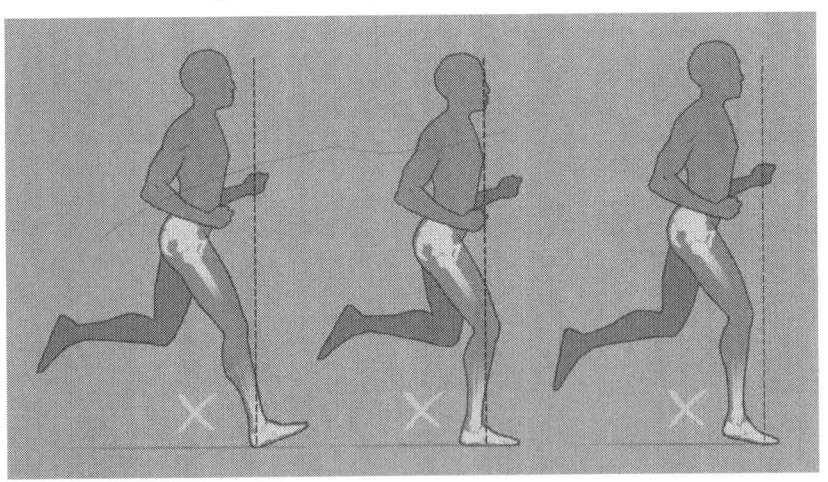

Illustration 1: *Heel (left), midfoot (middle), and forefoot (right) landing examples. All three landing examples are over-strides. In each case, the runner is leaning back as they land. This causes them to slow down.*

When most people talk about over striding, they think they are only doing this when they extend their stride length (i.e. the distance between landings) by stretching out. Actually, they are over-striding whenever their foot does not land under their hips. You can get away with this for years, even decades, with sheer determination. However, skeletal degeneration can occur, and you'll be prone to knee and hip replacements and back operations. The sinister aspect of this is that these symptoms are not always immediately apparent. Other factors that make it difficult to recognise the problems are 'chunky' shoes and strength training. The shoes cushion your feet but not the rest of your body. Strength training on the other hand allows you to cope with the impact on your body of poor technique, but this just delays the inevitable onset of injuries.

The 'heel-strike' over-stride

A heel-strike is always an over-stride. *Illustration 2* depicts a hard, decelerating heel-strike landing and the stress points (dark areas) as the body levers itself past the foot, which is inhibiting the runner's forwards motion. The initial impact (left figure) and then stress points (right figure) are a result of braking, balancing and supporting multiple times the body weight.

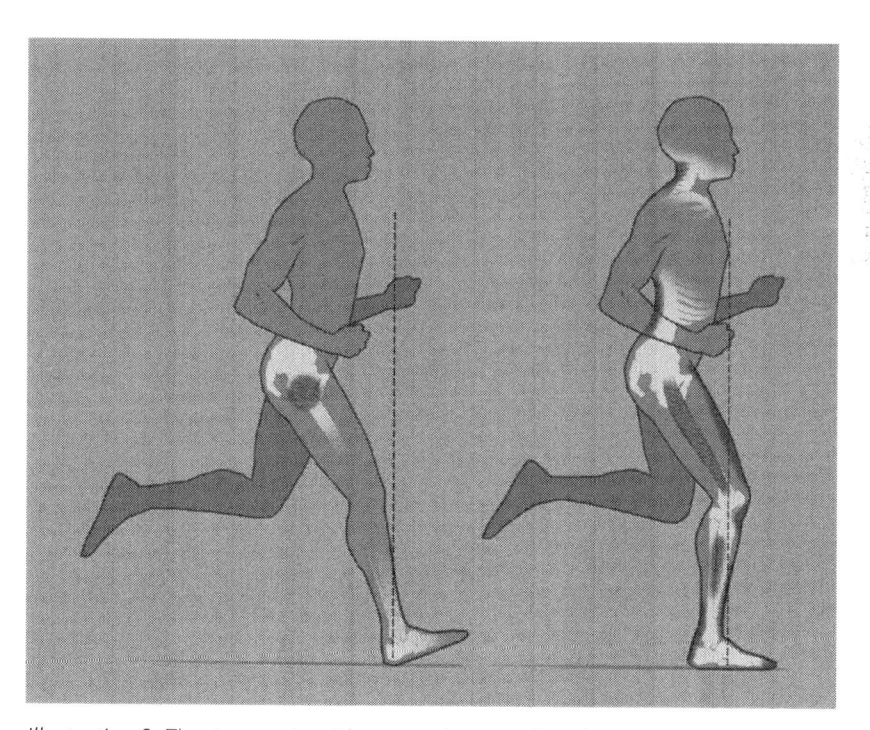

Illustration 2: The stress points (dark areas) caused by a heel-strike over-stride. The initial impact (left) and then stress points (right) are a result of braking, balancing and supporting multiple times the body weight.

Some light, long-legged, usually female, runners can manage a lighter heel-strike landing and a heel–toe rolling action with a good speed. They seem to suffer less injuries initially, but we often see them with serious hip problems as they get older.

The 'forefoot-strike' over-stride

A forefoot-strike is also an over-stride. *Illustration 3* shows the stress points on initial impact (left figure) of a fore-foot-strike and the stress points (right figure), which are a result of braking, balancing and supporting multiple times the body weight.

Some runners have heard that they should 'forefoot run' and they attempt to fix their technique by adjusting their landing. But, trying to force a particular foot 'strike' is not going to help, and is likely to cause injury.

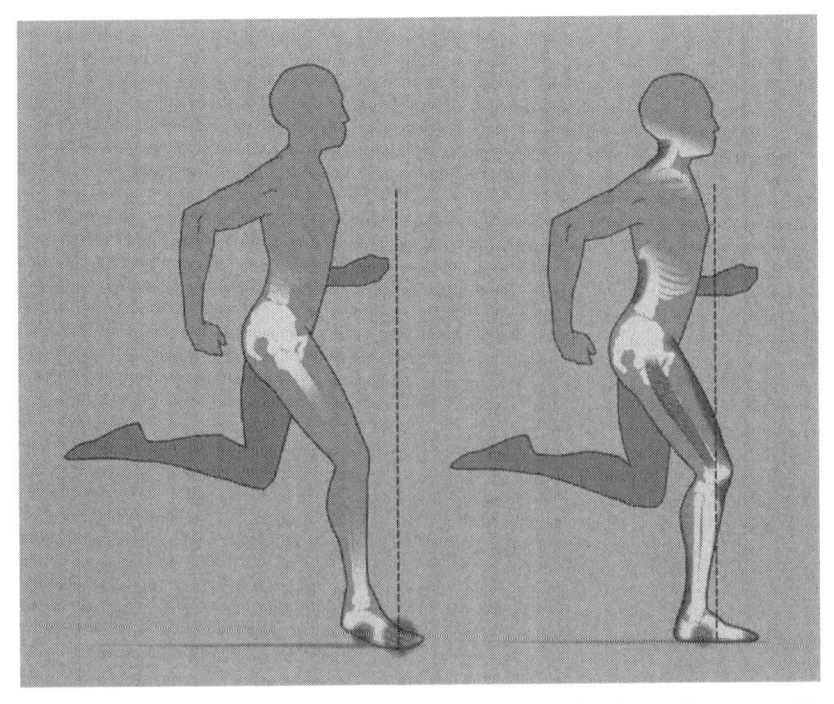

Illustration 3: *The stress points (dark areas) caused by a forefoot-strike over-stride. The initial impact (left) and then stress points (right) are a result of braking, balancing and supporting multiple times the body weight.*

The 'midfoot-strike' over-stride

The midfoot-strike over-stride (see *Illustration 1*, middle figure) is not as damaging as the other two because there is less stress on the feet. This over-stride problem often arises when people think that heel-striking and forefoot striking are wrong, and they attempt to change their foot-landing angle rather than trying to achieve a balanced landing.

You cannot cure over-striding by changing your foot strike.

1.2 How to check if you are over-striding

When you over-stride, your running suffers in many ways, but the good news is that this gives you many opportunities to recognise any flaws in your technique. When you do fix your over-stride, you will find that you can achieve great things. It's something the best runners think about at the most important moments. Mo Farah said, 'I was just digging in, digging in and making sure I didn't over-stride' when he ran a 54-second last lap to hold off Ibrahim Jeilan in the 10,000 metres World Championships in 2013. Top runners are always making sure that they don't fall into an over-stride.

If you run with poor form, you won't be running smoothly. Your harsh, uneven movements will not only give you away, but will be an indication of injuries waiting to happen. The lucky runners are those whose injuries or slow times cause them stop and think about what they are doing to themselves. We hope that is you.

A good way to check your running technique is to ask a friend to take a side-view video at constant speed and choose a frame where your foot has full pressure against the ground. This is the first of our ten OYF Rules that summarise the take-home messages of this book.

> **OYF Rule #1: Get a side-view video regularly**
>
> You might think your foot is already landing under your hips, but you will find that in most instances it certainly is not. The only way to identify the extent of your over-stride is to take a side-view video. A front or back-view video will not show the over-stride and are largely irrelevant.

> Ask a friend to take a video of you running at constant speed. Once you have the video, choose a frame where your foot has full pressure against the ground. Draw a vertical line through the centre of that ground-contact point. If your hips are behind the line, then you are leaning back and braking. Compare your results with *Illustration 18*, which shows perfectly aligned landing and the aligned take-off position that will produce it.
>
> Continue to take side-view videos regularly throughout your transition.

1.3 Recognising the signs of poor technique

There are several signs that point to poor running technique. These include: lack of speed, abrasions on the soles of your shoes, poor posture, upper-body rotation, over-pronation, hip-drop, tripping and repetitive stress. We discuss each of these in more detail below.

Lack of speed

If you are struggling to break five minutes per kilometre (eight minutes per mile), then this is a clear sign that your energy is not being well spent!

It is not because you are unfit or lack talent—it is the technique you are using, normally compounded by wearing thick, soft, unstable, angled shoes or orthotics. You will find more on this topic in Chapter 14, *Shoes—what you need to know* and in Appendix B, *For podiatrists—treating runners*.

Lack of speed is caused by braking unnecessarily—if your foot lands in front of your hips, it acts like a brake, regardless of which part of your foot strikes the ground first. You are leaning back and using up your energy as you lever your body past your foot.

Even if you are a beginner runner, it is not difficult to run at five minutes per kilometre within the first year of training. We have a friend who started running at the age of 65, just after retirement and, although running only short distances while he built strength, he was very soon running at almost 6 minutes per kilometre because he was running with good technique.

Abrasions on the soles of your shoes

If your shoe slips back as you take off, or forwards as you land, then you are braking and accelerating each stride, and your soles will show that your shoes wear accordingly (if you are running barefoot, this will result in blisters).

In bad cases, you can hear this sliding on landing, especially on grass or gravel and, in extreme cases, also on the pavement.

A good reason for wearing light shoes and doing an occasional barefoot session on a hard surface is that you will feel this happening and start to self-correct.

Once you are running well, even at quite high speeds, your foot will land at a speed close to zero and most force will be downward. There will be no need push forwards to regain lost speed. *Illustration 4* shows the difference.

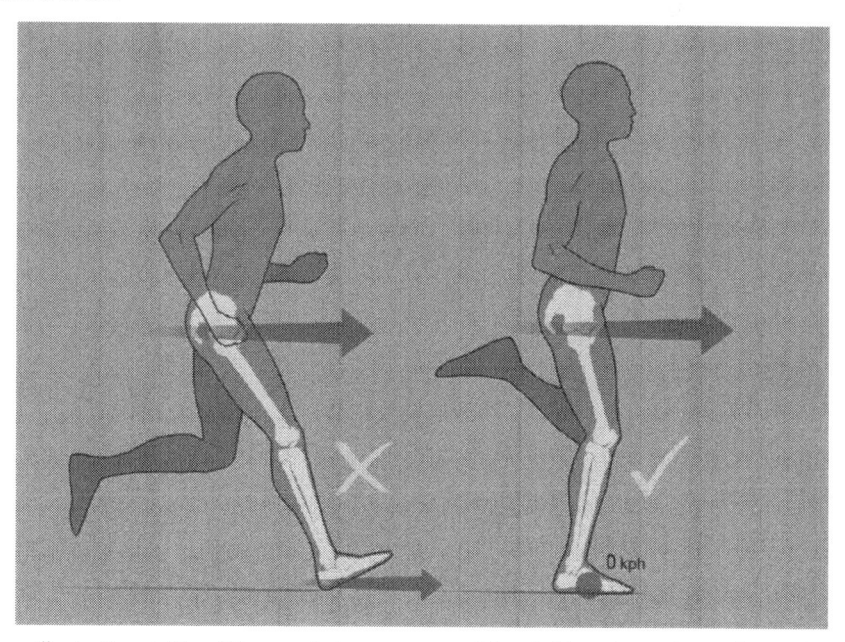

Illustration 4: The difference between over-striding (left) and running with good form (right).

When over-striding (left figure), the foot is moving forwards as it lands, causing you to brake. When running with good form (right figure), the foot is moving backwards just before it lands, which means there is hardly any braking and your body is vertically aligned, giving you full support and an immediate 'spring-assisted' take-off. Close to 0 kilometres per hour is the ideal foot-landing speed.

Most shoe retailers, manufacturers and podiatrists will probably tell you that you need to replace your shoes after, say, 800–1000 kilometres. One of the benefits of good technique and light shoes is that it significantly increases shoe life, simply because there is much less impact and less friction. We expect to wear out the uppers of our shoes before the soles.

Poor posture

If your foot is landing in front of your hips, the increased force and the lack of absorption by your legs causes your body to collapse at the waist. You won't engage your core muscles or your glutes (the gluteus medius, one of three gluteal muscles in the buttocks, which is responsible for hip stability and countering internal rotation of the thigh), and your posture will suffer as a consequence. You will develop a muscle imbalance between your quadriceps muscles (the four muscles that make up the thigh) and your glutes. This tends to lead to a curve in the lower back, often resulting in back and neck pain.

Don't bother working on core strength to fix this: if you land your foot in front of you at significant speed, you will collapse at the waist irrespective of how strong your core is!

Conversely, runners who consistently land near-vertically aligned, build postural strength from landing in this strong, stable position. This is a very important rule and the second OYF Rule. The rule will be further explained in Chapter 3, and also in Chapter 15, *How to get a hot runner's body*.

OYF Rule #2: Stand and land aligned

The aim is for your spine to be vertical, which means you will engage the postural muscles of your stomach (abdominals), back (erector spinae) and bottom (gluteals). You should be in this upright stance whenever you are standing, walking or running and it can only be achieved by wearing thin, flat, flexible shoes. When running, you can only land aligned if you have such shoes.

> By following this rule, you will build up all your muscles in the right proportions—calves, glutes, back, stomach, neck—every muscle you use will build as required. If you have spent decades in shoes that are raised up at the heel, then your muscles will have developed (and under-developed) to accommodate your non-vertical stance, and it will take some time for your body to re-adjust.

Upper-body rotation

Illustration 5 shows that upper-body rotation (top arrow) is a counter-rotation using the arms or shoulders necessary to balance lower-body rotation (bottom arrow) caused by over-striding.

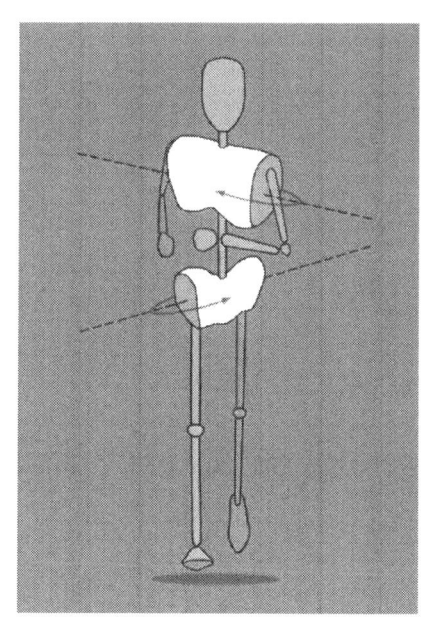

Illustration 5: *Lower-body rotation (bottom arrow) and upper-body counter-rotation (top arrow) caused by over-striding.*

To feel how this works, try standing still and swinging your arms across your body. You will feel your hips counter-rotating. If you try it when running, you will feel your leg action adjusting to compensate. To see how much your shoulders are rotating while running, try running for a few metres with your hands held together behind your back. This will accentuate any excess shoulder rotation so that you can start to correct it.

A relaxed arm swing should be all you need to counter any lower-body rotation at low to moderate speeds (you will be running at these speeds most of the time). At high speed, you can expect a gentle, graceful shoulder rotation.

Over-pronation

If you have foot and lower-leg injuries, you may over-pronate when you run. Pronation and supination are the rolling movements of the foot during walking and running. Pronation is where the foot rolls inward towards the inner edge of the sole and it is vital for absorbing landing forces and adapting to uneven surfaces. Supination is the opposite, where the foot rolls outward, acting as a rigid lever to push off for power.

Whether walking or running, your anatomy dictates that you land in a slightly supinated position. Your foot then pronates until your hips are above your foot and your whole foot provides full support.

It then supinates again as you leave the ground. Pronation is a necessary part of your suspension and will be just right when you run well.

If you over-pronate, it is because you over-stride. This is the third OYF Rule (see OYF Rule #3 below). You should not try to prevent over-pronation with supportive shoes or orthotics.

When you over-pronate, you are spending more time on the ground waiting for your hips to move over your foot and this greatly increases the rotational forces of pronation, resulting in foot and lower-leg injuries such as:

- stress fracture of metatarsal heads
- Achilles tendonitis or tendinosis
- plantar fasciitis and heel spurs
- posterior tibial tendonitis
- peroneal tendonitis
- shin splints, anterior or posterior
- stress fracture of the tibia (shin bone) or fibula (the thin bone that runs to the outside of the shin bone).

These injuries are discussed in more detail in Chapter 2, *Poor technique causes injuries*.

> ## OYF Rule #3: Over-pronation is a symptom of over-striding
>
> Your foot pronates throughout the whole landing. When you over-stride, landing takes much longer than normal and this causes over-pronation.
>
> Blocking pronation (the foot rolling inward on landing) with supportive shoes or orthotics will force you to continue to damage your body with high-impact landings, and put undue stress across your whole body.
>
> By following Keith's Lessons in this book, you will reduce any over-pronation you have by decreasing your over-stride. Being upright (OYF Rule #2) will strengthen your feet and your glutes and make sure over-pronation is never a problem again.

Hip-drop

If you over-stride, you will probably find that the unsupported side of your hips drops as you land. This is because you are hitting the ground with more force, and you have to balance on one leg for longer than you should. Your medical professional might suggest hip-hitching or glute-strengthening exercises and these will certainly do no harm. However, if you don't fix your over-stride, when you resume running, injury is very likely. With good running form, your glutes and your whole core will start to be used every landing and your hip-drop will vanish.

Tripping

Tripping is a very obvious symptom of over-striding; if your foot goes ahead of your body close to the ground, it can easily collide with low-lying obstacles. In good running, the foot is pulled up off the ground by the hips and is high above any obstacles when it is going forwards. When you run well, tripping is very difficult, even on rough ground.

Repetitive stress

A typical over-strider will take at least 160 steps per minute, so they repeat their stressful landings almost 10 000 times each hour they run. This is why running injuries are so common!

When your foot lands in front of your body, your body has to catch up with your foot before you can take off again. During this time, your quadriceps, your hip flexors and your iliotibial bands (the fibrous sheath down the outside of the thigh, connecting the hip to the knee) are supporting and stabilising your upper body with a loading equivalent to many times your body weight. This load increases dramatically as you speed up. Knee and iliotibial band problems can take a long time to appear due to the strength of the muscles and bones in your upper leg. However, the excessive stress will eventually cause a breakdown.

If you frequently have to stretch your quads or hip flexors, or if you have to roll out your iliotibial bands, then you are overusing them.

1.4 Run, don't walk

One way of thinking about the differences between good technique and poor technique is to compare the extremes of skilful race walking and skilful race running. The following comparison is useful for many runners to think about while they are working on their technique.

Race walkers must have one foot on the ground all the time, or risk disqualification, and therefore all their stride length comes from stretching their legs out along the ground. On the other hand, in good runners the stride length comes from being airborne at speed, and the leg action is centred on the nature of the ground contact, not on stretching out.

Most runners have varying degrees of race walking in their running technique. However, efficient runners do not. They do not stretch forwards at all; they use their legs for support and to lift their body away from the ground. They hardly have to push forwards because they hardly slow down. They bounce and fly, our fourth OYF Rule.

> ### OYF Rule #4: Bounce and fly
>
> Once you have mastered good running technique, you will naturally run faster and you will be surprised that your training times improve with no extra effort.
>
> By simply concentrating on a balanced landing, you will continually reduce your braking and at the same time make yourself strong in the right places. This will make you land well and close to vertically aligned, with all your postural muscles naturally engaged. Then, once landed, the elasticity in your feet and legs will bounce you to a long stride and make you run faster.

Your objective is to be in the air as much as possible, but with the least effort. Improve your technique and you will reduce your over-stride and increase your stride length too!

Long legs are a limited advantage

Runners with long legs are able to get a long stride and run quickly by extending their long legs in front of them instead of getting airborne. However, this is inefficient and there is a very high risk of injury.

We know a number of fast female runners in this category who have suffered multiple lower-leg stress fractures and hip damage, which sometimes resulted in early hip-replacement operations.

It is frustrating to read advertisements for popular shoes that promote this technique by advertising a 'smooth heel-to-toe action'. Running with good technique will produce better results. We say 'Spring, don't swing', and that is our fifth OYF Rule.

OYF Rule #5: Spring, don't swing

By 'spring, don't swing' we mean do not swing your legs, or try to lift your knees or feet.

The 'spring' part comes from the elastic energy in an unrestricted foot and Achilles tendon, and is the result of landing balanced. The spring produces an immediate take-off in a slightly more forwards direction. In efficient running, getting airborne is natural and seems effortless (OYF Rule #4).

The more you need to push off when at constant speed, the more you will have braked upon landing. However, the best runners have very little 'drive': they quickly 'bounce' their body off their whole foot after landing near-vertically aligned with minimal braking.

CHAPTER 2
POOR TECHNIQUE CAUSES INJURIES

Keith Bateman and Heidi Jones

As we showed in Chapter 1, flaws in your technique direct large forces to certain parts of your body, and it is these parts that hurt when you run, or after running, and ultimately become injured. The main flaw is over-striding, which causes unbalanced high-impact landings. As a general principle, if you notice that one part of your body is stressed more than others, we suggest that you look at your running technique.

If you continue to run with poor technique you will eventually get injured, and there is a good correlation between the way you run and the injuries you incur. For example, if you have a forefoot-strike over-stride, you are in great danger of injuring your feet as well as suffering Achilles tendonitis, ankle and knee pain. If you have a heel-strike over-stride, you are likely to suffer from iliotibial band, knee, hip and back pain.

In this chapter, we detail the main causes of common running injuries so that you can use this information to identify the technique fault that has caused your injury. We first look at injuries to the feet, and then at injuries to the rest of the body. Finally, we discuss how attempts to alleviate some of these problems with external aids are only treating the symptom, and not the cause.

2.1 Injuries to the feet

Illustration 6 shows the symptoms of injuries in the main parts of the foot that can result from over-striding. We discuss these injuries in the following sections.

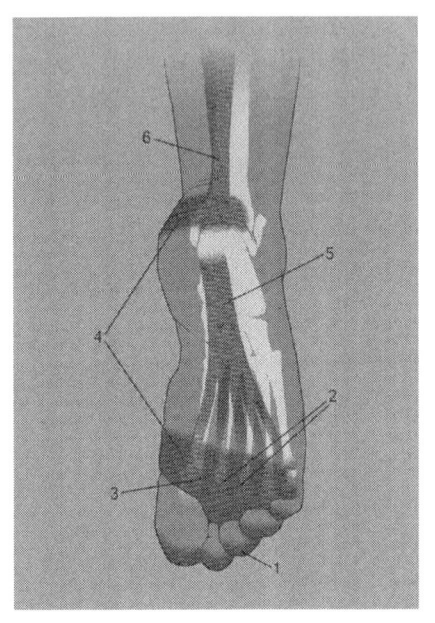

Illustration 6: Location of symptoms of over-striding in the foot. 1. Damaged toes, 2. Metatarsal head stress fracture, 3. Forefoot soreness (metatarsalgia and burning feet), 4. Blisters, 5. Plantar fasciitis, 6. Achilles tendonitis or tendinosis.

Damaged toes

Injuries to the toe nails and on the end or bottom of the toes (*Illustration 6.1*) are usually caused by your toes pushing into the front of your shoe. Injuries include: bruised toes, calluses on the ends of your toes, blood under your toe nails, thickened or lost toe nails.

These injuries happen when you brake and your foot moves forwards, pressing on the front of the shoe. Some runners clench their toes in their shoes and this can have a similar effect. Barefoot runners who over-stride badly will often suffer blisters under their toes, as they push off hard each take-off.

Metatarsal head stress fracture

A metatarsal head fracture (*Illustration 6.2*) or march fracture is caused by rotational forces and excessive strain associated with excessive pronation.

Landing on the toes produces this injury, as does slapping the ground after a heel-strike landing. This injury is most common in the second and third metatarsals.

Forefoot soreness

Problems under the ball of the foot (*Illustration 6.3*) include two different injuries: metatarsalgia and burning feet. Metatarsalgia is caused by the foot striking the ground. A burning sensation in the feet is caused by the shearing force as the foot slips on landing.

Forefoot soreness is a common symptom with people who forefoot-strike. It is particularly common when wearing very thin shoes and landing on the forefoot alone, and often looks like 'prancing' or a horse doing dressage.

Shoes with a 'turned-up' toe box and a 'drop' contribute to metatarsalgia. The drop of the shoe, also referred to as the heel-to-toe drop, is a measure of how much taller the heel is than the forefoot (see also Chapter 14, *Shoes—what you need to know*). This type of shoe holds the feet in a position where the metatarsal heads are exposed, leaving the feet susceptible to injury. At the same time, the heel–toe running action—which this type of shoe induces—forces excess pressure onto the ball of the foot.

Blisters

Blisters on the back of the heel or under the forefoot (*Illustration 6.4*) arise when your foot is moving in relation to your shoe.

This is caused by a stiff shoe, or skin shearing due to the constant braking and acceleration associated with over-striding. Barefoot runners might get blisters under the forefoot from skin shearing if their technique isn't good.

Plantar fasciitis

The plantar fascia (*Illustration 6.5*) is the thick fibrous band on the bottom of the foot running from the heel to the five toes.

Plantar fasciitis is a common, painful disorder affecting the bottom of the heel and the underside of the foot. It is caused by increased strain on the plantar fascia at its origin. Stiff shoes with raised heels and turned-up toe boxes are major contributors (see *Illustration 7*).

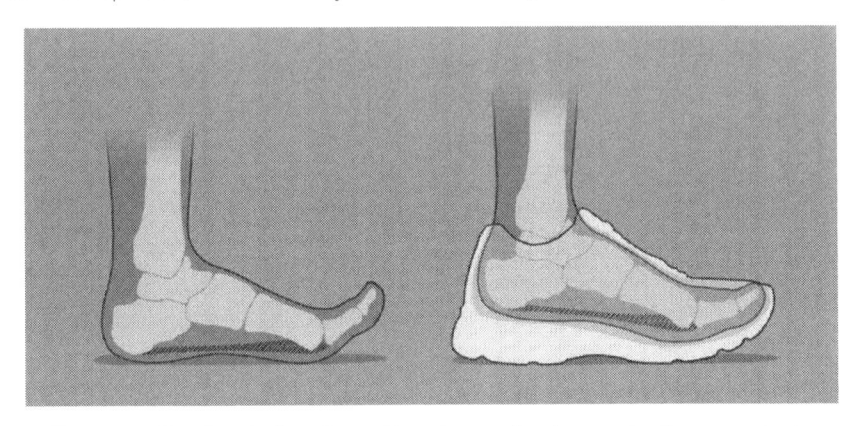

Illustration 7: *Left. Windlass Stress Test that podiatrists use to diagnose plantar fasciitis. It involves stressing the plantar fascia (dark area). Right. Most shoes put your foot in the Windlass Stress Test stressed position all the time, even when standing. They also open up and load the metatarsal joints, exposing them to injury.*

Heidi, in her capacity as a podiatrist, sees a big correlation between chunky shoes and plantar fasciitis, even in non-runners. It is of course important that your running technique does not stress your plantar fascia either. 'Toe-running', where the runner lands heavily, or only on their toes, will cause such stress.

Achilles tendonitis and tendinosis

The Achilles tendon (*Illustration 6.6*) is the tendon that connects the calf muscles (gastrocnemius and soleus, which form the bulge on the back of the lower leg) to the heel bone. It is the thickest tendon in the human body.

Achilles tendonitis is an inflammation of the Achilles tendon. Achilles tendinosis is the chronic condition where there is thickening and scar tissue within the Achilles tendon if the Achilles tendonitis is not properly rehabilitated.

When over-striding, the increased time the foot is on the ground and the accompanying excessive pronation result in increased strain and unnatural torque placed on the Achilles tendon. Toe-running often produces this injury. Many children also suffer 'growing pains' in this area (Sever's disease). Heavily cushioned shoes make the situation worse.

Heidi sees a big correlation between thick-soled, spongy shoes and Achilles tendonitis, even in non-runners.

2.2 Injuries to the rest of the body

Illustration 8 shows symptoms of injuries across the body that can result from over-striding. We discuss these injuries in the following sections.

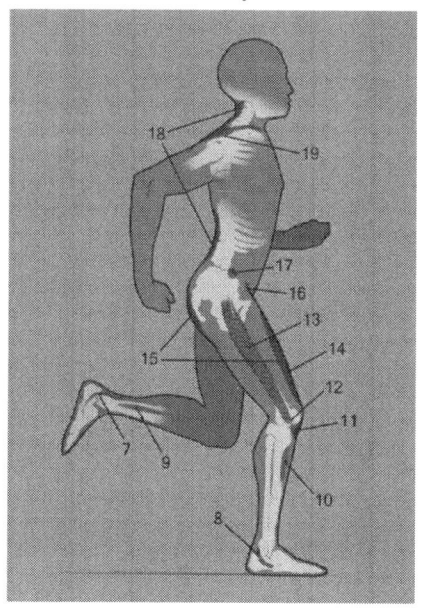

Illustration 8: Location of symptoms of over-striding across the body (numbering continues from symptoms listed in Illustration 6). 7. Posterior tibial tendonitis, 8. Peroneal tendonitis, 9. Posterior shin splints, 10. Anterior shin splints, 11. Runner's knee, 12. Iliotibial band friction syndrome, 13. Tight iliotibial band, 14. Tight quads, 15 Muscle imbalance—strong quads and weak glutes, 16. Hip flexor pain, 17. Bursitis of the hip, 18. Back or neck tension, 19. Shoulder tension.

Posterior tibial tendonitis

Posterior tibial tendonitis (*Illustration 8.7*) occurs when the posterior tibial tendon becomes inflamed or torn.

It includes pain behind and under the inside of the ankle bone and is due to excessive pronation from over-striding.

As the foot lands, it will pronate, and continue to pronate until the hips have moved over the foot. When over-striding, this increases time on the ground, which causes the tendon to be overused and over-stretched. Long-term use of orthotics will weaken the posterior tibial tendon due to its continued support.

Peroneal tendonitis

Peroneal tendonitis (*Illustration 8.8*) occurs when the peroneal tendon has become inflamed or torn. Pain behind and under the outside of the ankle bone is due to excessive pronation from over-striding.

Thick, spongy shoes and shoes with different density materials on the sole appear to be a major contributing factor to peroneal tendonitis by causing the foot to ricochet from pronation to supination.

Posterior shin splints

Posterior shin splints, also called medial tibial stress syndrome (*Illustration 8.9*), is pain felt along the back-inside of your shin bone, where the tibialis posterior muscle is attached. The pain is caused by overusing the stabilising muscles of the lower leg due to excessive pronation.

The tibialis posterior is the key stabilising muscle of the lower leg that attaches to the arch of the foot. It is located at the back and to the inside of the shin bone (tibia). This muscle supports the medial longitudinal arch of the foot (the instep or main arch). It assists with plantarflexion (stretching away from the shin, i.e. pointing) of the foot and with inversion (sole arcing inwards). This combined action is called supination.

When over-striding, the tibialis posterior muscle gets overused due to the increased time the foot is on the ground waiting for the hips to move over the foot (excessive pronation). These increased rotational forces are made worse by wearing orthotics or stiff shoes.

If you do not stop running when you have this injury, you may sustain a stress fracture of the tibia (see below).

Anterior shin splints

The tibialis anterior (*Illustration 8.10*) is the stabilising muscle at the front outside of the shin that attaches to the foot. It both dorsiflexes (foot pointing to shin) and inverts the foot (sole arcing inwards).

The tibialis anterior muscle decelerates the foot during heel-strike; thus it gets over-worked when doing this, especially when running downhill. This injury is very common with raised-heel, flared sole, stiff, chunky shoes.

If you do not stop running when you have this injury, you may sustain a stress fracture of the fibula (see below).

Heidi has seen runners suffering from chronic anterior shin splints who have been misdiagnosed with compartment syndrome. They have undergone surgery only to suffer from shin splints again when resuming running.

Compartment syndrome occurs when there is swelling or bleeding within a compartment of the muscle; for example, front of the shin (tibialis anterior).

Stress fracture of the tibia or fibula

Stress fractures of the tibia or fibula are also caused by excessive pronation and usually occur in runners with supportive shoes or orthotics. They are often preceded by shin splints that has been left untreated.

Runner's knee

Runner's knee or chondromalacia patellae is a condition where the cartilage on the under-surface of the kneecap (patella) deteriorates and softens.

Runner's knee is one of the most common causes of pain under or below the kneecap (*Illustration 8.11*). The pain is caused by irritation and inflammation where the knee cap slides over the lower end of the thighbone. It usually arises after a running session, gradually gets worse following subsequent sessions, and is more painful when going up and down stairs.

The injury is most commonly caused by a quadriceps muscle imbalance when over-striding during running, which is causing a lateral pull on the kneecap. This imbalance is caused by the lateral forces on your iliotibial band and quadriceps muscles while you lean back and have to balance as you land. Repeating this action thousands of times per leg per hour leads to the injury.

There is a high correlation between runner's knee and weak glutes, and that fits with the fact that if you over-stride your glutes don't work, and your quads get overused.

Tight quadriceps muscles

Tight quadriceps (*Illustration 8.14*) is caused by excessive use of these muscles to support the knee and upper body when landing with the foot ahead of the hips.

Ask yourself whether you are running tall and getting a rebound from your landings (which is good), or whether you are 'squatting' each time you land and dissipating your energy into your quadriceps (which is bad).

Tight iliotibial band

The iliotibial band is the fibrous sheath down the outside of the thigh, connecting the hip to the knee (*Illustration 8.13*).

When over-striding, you need to use your iliotibial bands to continually stabilise your torso. This means you are landing in an unbalanced, backwards-leaning position (hips behind your foot, collapsing at the waist) and repeating this thousands of times per leg per hour.

Pain in the iliotibial band is made worse by running on uneven ground and running downhill. In our experience this is 100% fixable by changing your technique, and so far Keith has achieved this for all his clients in one session.

Iliotibial band friction syndrome

Increased flexion of the knee joint due to collapsing into a squat position during over-striding can also cause irritation where the iliotibial band crosses over the outside of the knee (*Illustration 8.12*).

Muscle imbalance

Having strong quads and weak glutes (*Illustration 8.15*) is caused by over-striding, which makes you collapse at the waist upon landing. In this squat position you use your quads almost exclusively and hardly use your glutes. You can rectify this imbalance with specific strengthening exercises, but unless you amend your technique, the imbalance will return.

Raising the heel of a shoe switches off the glutes, so check the shoes you wear for every activity (see also OYF Rule #2).

Good technique will ensure balanced muscle use. If you have been running for a few months, and your butt and stomach muscles have not started to tighten up, then you are not landing balanced. Landing balanced (with your foot under your hips) requires those muscles to be used over 10,000 times per hour. Run well and you will get a good runner's body in less time than you might expect (see Chapter 15, *How to get a hot runner's body*).

Hip pain

Hip pain includes pain in the hip flexors (at the front) and bursitis of the hip (on the bone).

Hip flexor pain (*Illustration 8.16*) is caused by excessive use of this muscle due to foot-lifting and leg-swinging, which makes your foot land in front of you. This dramatically increases the force on your hip flexors as your hips drop towards the ground each time you land in a semi-squat position.

Bursitis of the hip (*Illustration 8.17*) is inflammation of the small cushioning sac located where the tendons pass over the hip bone. It is caused by friction, which itself is caused by the repetitive trauma of excessive force going up the skeleton and by landing in a crouched position.

Upper-body pain

Upper-body pain is caused by excessive impact forces, and deceleration and acceleration, together with a lack of spring in your legs. It results in back or neck pain and shoulder pain.

Tension in the lower back and the neck (*Illustration 8.18*) is from not landing vertically aligned, combined with the stop–start action of over-striding. You can often see a runner's head move forwards and back each landing and take-off as they brake and accelerate. You might also notice their body makes a 'C' shape when viewed from the side.

Excessive tension in your shoulders (*Illustration 8.19*) is due to a heavy landing and a lack of suspension in your legs. Once your landings are soft and smooth, the tension will be relieved. Heidi suffered from this for 25 years before changing her technique.

2.3 Dealing with injuries

Many runners try to use bandages, tape, straps, orthotics and injections as quick fixes for their running injuries. These short-term measures only mask a problem and result in treating symptoms and not causes.

If you need support, you are injured or weak, or both. Avoiding the issue does not address the problem and is likely to create an injury elsewhere. It is a recipe for disaster (see *Illustration 9*).

Your medical practitioner might be treating your symptoms, such as weak glutes, over-pronation, hip-drop, iliotibial band soreness, and so on. But, if you fix the cause by changing your technique, these symptoms can be fixed quickly and permanently. This is our sixth OYF Rule.

> ### OYF Rule #6: Fix the problem not the symptom
>
> There is only one thing you need to fix in running: your over-stride.
>
> Simply by reducing this, you will learn to land more balanced and you will start to fix everything else. This is because almost all injuries, and lack of speed, are due to your foot landing too far in front of you.
>
> Trying to fix the symptom of over-striding with artificial supports, orthotics, 'special' shoes and so on, will just obscure the problem, allowing you to run badly for longer. You will continue to suffer.

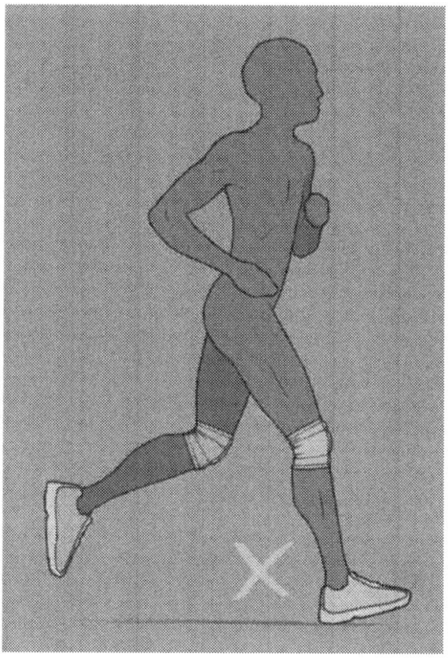

Illustration 9: This illustration, taken from a real picture of an over-striding runner, shows how runners try to stop knee pain so they can run without pain. This is a recipe for disaster. Knee supports merely allow runners to continue pounding their body until a more serious injury incapacitates them! We predict this runner will develop hip flexor pain, a lower-leg stress fracture or will need knee or hip surgery at a young age.

Our advice, which in our experience always works, is:

- Do not believe the 'no pain, no gain' philosophy. If you have prolonged pain, you will not gain.
- Rest. This is nature's greatest healer. And pain is nature's messenger.
- Follow *Heidi's Strengthening Program* (Chapter 11).
- Ditch any chunky shoes and walk and run in thin, flat, flexible shoes, or no shoes.
- Re-learn how to run properly.
- Allow the new muscle groups to naturally build up.

Follow these principles and hopefully you will run until you are 100 or beyond—we intend to!

CHAPTER 3
GOOD TECHNIQUE—HOW IT WORKS

Keith Bateman

Good technique is the same for everyone. We are born with it; just watch children running barefoot at the beach, where they run very well, on any surface. Unfortunately, as adults, we tend to lose this natural ability with our busy lifestyle and we have to re-train ourselves into running with good form. To run well you need to be strong both mentally and physically. The good news is that, as you follow the principles of OYF Running and Keith's Lessons, you will automatically build this physical strength and gain the mental confidence you require to be a good runner. Do not worry about so-called 'abnormalities' you might have. If you were born with them, your body will have adjusted well, and if you have acquired them from making the wrong movements, then the lessons and exercises in this book should rectify this too.

Running combines two distinct actions. There is the near-continuous forwards momentum of your body in combination with the stop–start contact of your foot with the ground. The art of good running is to coordinate these and create a fluid and efficient running motion. Great runners like Haile Gebrselassie, Steve Ovett, Mo Farah and Zola Budd all run in a similar relaxed manner: they are not straining, they are fluid and flying, and this is how you can run too. It is how all humans should run.

What we have described above, is what we see as the most efficient technique for running—something that all humans would naturally do if they continued running from childhood without interruption and were not influenced by shoes. It is a technique that fixes all the people we see, and we have no doubt it is what all runners should aim for.

However, there are some top-performing runners who, over the years, have shown they can land their foot considerably in front of their hips and use sheer power to maintain a good speed. Landing the foot well in front of the body *is* a slowing action that requires great strength, especially in the quadriceps. However, the more powerful take-off that is made possible by being on the ground longer gives them an extended stride length. The downside of this is that, as well as requiring very strong quads and hip flexors, it has greater potential for knee and iliotibial band injuries, and greatly reduces the ability to sprint. There is also a high chance of hip injuries. It boggles our mind to think how much faster these runners could go if they amended their technique.

In this chapter, we look at how good technique works in three aspects of the running action—landing, take-off and accelerating—which are then covered in more depth in the first three lessons.

3.1 Landing

I have started with landings because this is the easiest phase of the running action to learn, and it sets you up for your take-offs.

Balanced landing

The most important aspect of a balanced landing is to be as near as possible to being vertically aligned: your foot should be under your hips once you have fully landed (see *Illustration 10*).

To observe your landing, making a side-view video of you running at constant speed (OYF Rule #1) is important. The side-view video will help you recognise how much you are over-striding; that is, how much you are leaning backwards as you land. Keith's Lessons (Chapters 5 to 10) will help you correct this error and, as you move towards a balanced landing, you will find that everything else in your running action starts to fall into place.

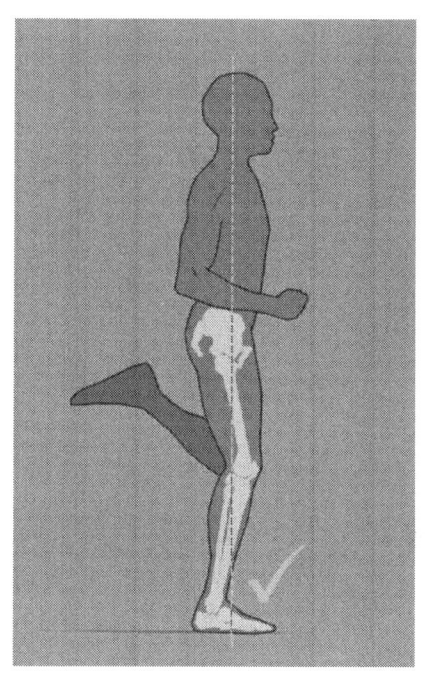

Illustration 10: Balanced landing. Hips above foot—landing vertically aligned.

If you land balanced, your running will become a continuous flowing action rather than a series of separate movements. You will find that you:

- run smoother and more relaxed
- use your energy supplies more efficiently
- maintain your speed
- get the best possible rebound
- dramatically reduce the impact of your landing
- minimise muscle stress and thus reduce your chances of injury
- are flexible in all directions and thus ready for obstacles or sudden direction changes
- find that most other problems in your running will be fixed
- use your muscles rather than your skeleton and therefore burn more fat (natural ketosis)—muscular strength is a big predictor of future good health.

Natural foot action

Your landing should be a natural action. We will describe this in detail so that you understand what's required to correct any errors that might have crept into your running. It is difficult to get an accurate picture of this complicated action as there is a lot of interaction between its components.

During each landing, the foot is in contact with the ground for milliseconds and a lot happens in this very short time. The landing is further complicated by the continuing forwards motion of the body, which prolongs the foot contact with the ground. There are two simultaneous motions of the foot:

- **The side-to-side pronation–supination action.**
  The inward-rolling motion (pronation) starts as the foot touches the ground in a slightly supinated position. This enables you to absorb the impact of landing and adapt to uneven surfaces. The outward-rolling motion (supination) locks the midfoot on take-off, making it a rigid lever for propulsion. In efficient running, this pronation–supination action is almost instantaneous, as the foot contacts the ground, fully lands, and rebounds.

- **The front–back action, which is a forefoot-wholefoot-forefoot action.**
  This motion distributes the load and provides most of the elastic energy (via the Achilles tendon and calf muscle) for a strong take-off. When the hips have caught up with the foot, the foot is 'fully loaded' and ready to spring.

Illustrations 11 and *12* give a side and front view of these two simultaneous actions in a balanced landing.

Illustration 11 shows the start of the landing (i.e. before fully landing), where your foot touches lightly in front of your hips in a slightly supinated position. *Illustration 12* shows the position of your body immediately after that, when completing the landing, where your foot fully lands under your hips.

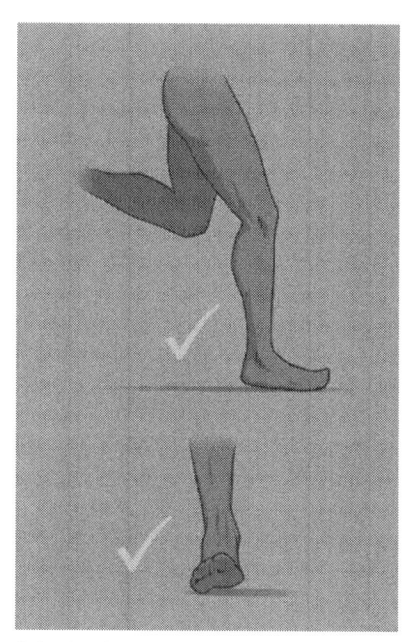

Illustration 11: Start of the landing (i.e. before fully landing). In a balanced landing, your foot will touch lightly in front of your hips in a slightly supinated position. Do not try to land like this—it will happen naturally once you learn to land balanced.

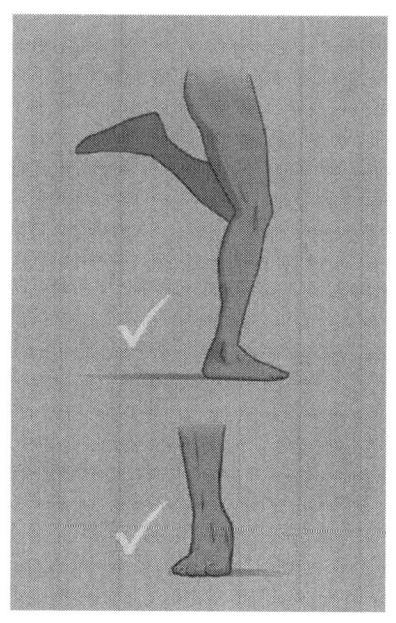

Illustration 12: Completed landing. In a balanced landing, when completed, your foot will fully land when it is under your hips. Do not try to land like this—it will happen naturally once you learn to land balanced.

If you land incorrectly, you will not be vertically aligned (see *Illustration 13* below) and you will not benefit from the spring off the ground and the longer stride length this gives you. The positive rebound effect is greatly reduced, if not eliminated, if you over-stride, whether it is a forefoot-, midfoot- or heel-strike over-stride, as shown in *Illustration 14*.

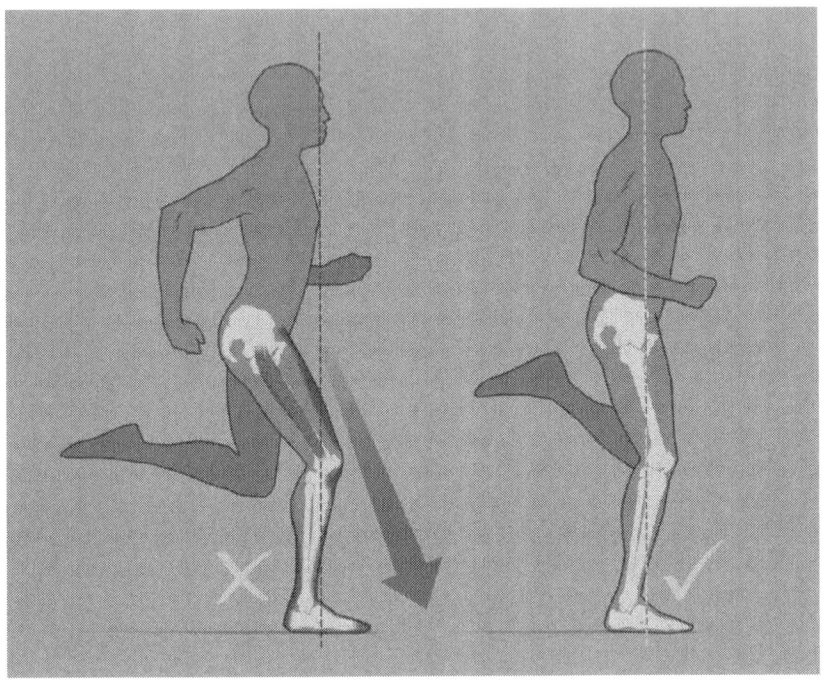

Illustration 13: Over-striding (left) means you are pushing against your direction of travel and increasing stress (dark areas) on certain parts of your body. The nearer you are to vertical (right) when landing, the less force there is on your body and the more evenly that force is distributed.

3.2 Take-off

When we say 'take-off', we are referring to leaving the ground after a landing. Your initial take-off from a stationary position is also very important, as it sets the trend for the rest of your run, but we cover this as a special case of acceleration in Section 3.3 below.

The take-off can be described in two parts. Firstly, the spring effect, which is achieved by landing your whole foot under your hips; and secondly, the push off the front of your forefoot to accelerate. A good runner will start their take-off from their vertically-aligned landing, which ensures that their foot is flat on the ground. Their body will rebound off the ground mostly off the whole foot, with the forefoot providing only a very small extra push.

If your foot lands in front (*Illustration 14*, left figure), you decelerate, absorb the shock of landing and have to push forwards to replace the speed you have just lost. However, if you land balanced, vertically aligned (*Illustration 14*, right figure), your legs then act as a spring, greatly reducing the effort required to leave the ground and reducing the necessity to push forwards. You can see dogs, large and small, using their legs in a similar way as they spring along a pavement, their ears flopping up and down as they 'bounce' down the street.

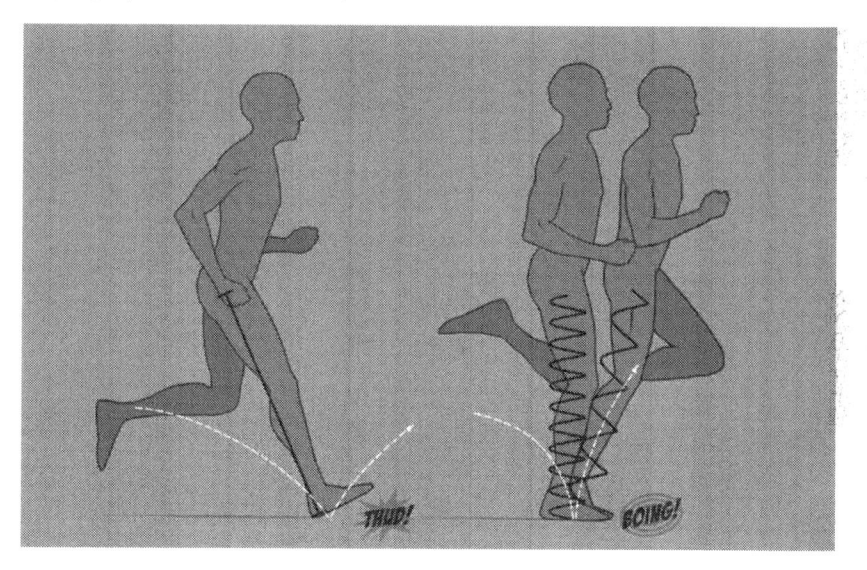

Illustration 14: High-impact over-stride (left) compared to a balanced, spring-loaded landing (right).

We will practice this type of landing in Chapter 5, *Lesson One: Landing*.

The better the runner, the less they will need to push off their forefoot to maintain a constant speed. A runner with poor form will land leaning backwards, absorb the extra impact and then have to push forwards off their forefoot or toes to accelerate.

A good way of checking your own landing and take-off is to run on firm sand and see what sort of imprint you leave in the sand when running at a constant speed. *Illustration* 15 shows an example of a good, smooth footprint, a sign of efficient running, next to a bad footprint left by an inefficient runner.

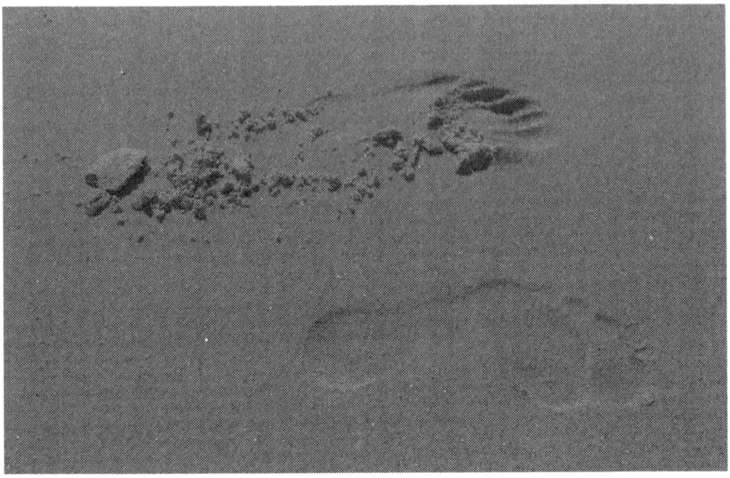

Illustration 15: Samples of bad (top) and good (bottom) footprints. A smooth footprint is a sign of efficient running (of not having to push forwards each step). Photo by Stuart Greaves.

Hips pull the foot

As you leave the ground, your hips continue to travel ahead of your partially grounded foot. We say, 'Hips first—your foot will follow' because this helps to combat over-striding. This is our seventh OYF Rule.

> ### OYF Rule #7: Hips first—your foot will follow
>
> The majority of runners lift or swing their legs forwards, which causes their hips to be behind their foot when they land. The way of overcoming this problem is to 're-program' your brain to focus on your back foot catching up with your hips, rather than advancing your front foot.
>
> The position you are looking for once you have fully landed is the position in the middle: neither leaning forwards or back. Don't make the mistake of pushing your hips forwards—just leave your foot on the ground and let your hips freely move ahead.

> Using a side-view video (OYF Rule #1), compare your results with *Illustration 18*, which shows perfectly aligned landing and the aligned take-off position that will produce it. To keep a check on your progress and to make sure you are running with good form, continue to take a side-view video regularly.

Most runners fall into the trap of advancing their foot so that it lands in front of them. *Illustration 16* shows that if you try to extend your stride length by advancing your foot, it will be in front when you land. Thinking about the foot following helps to overcome this error.

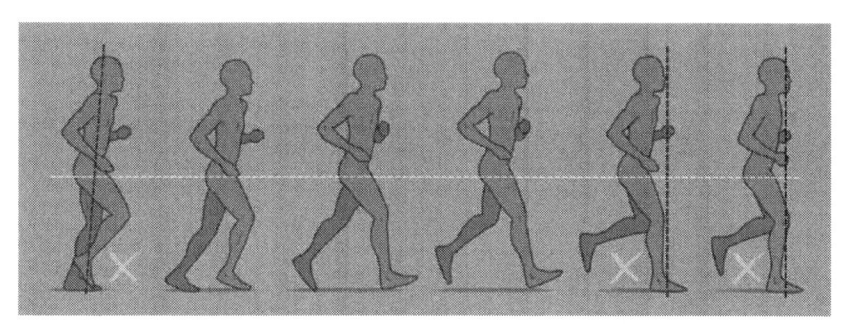

Illustration 16: *If you try to extend your stride length by advancing your foot it will be in front when you land. Notice the runner is barely getting off the ground.*

A similar fault is to lift the knee to increase your stride length, as in *Illustration 17*. This wastes even more energy—as the leg is a very heavy part of the body—and it also moves the foot ahead causing an over-stride.

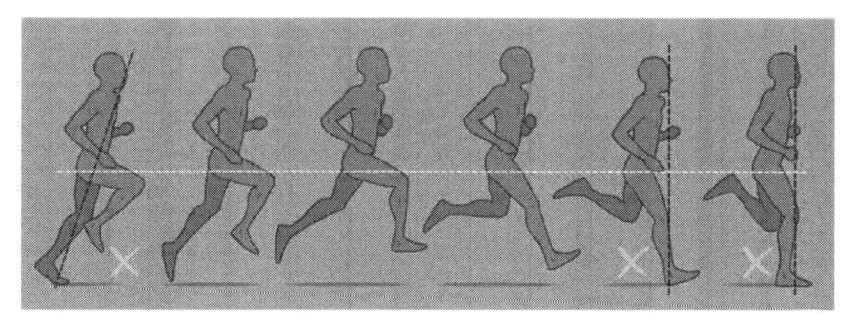

Illustration 17: *Trying to increase your stride length by lifting your knee is also advancing your foot and 'walking' forwards.*

Illustration 18 shows that, when running efficiently, your heel will move away from the ground naturally as you complete your take-off and leave the ground.

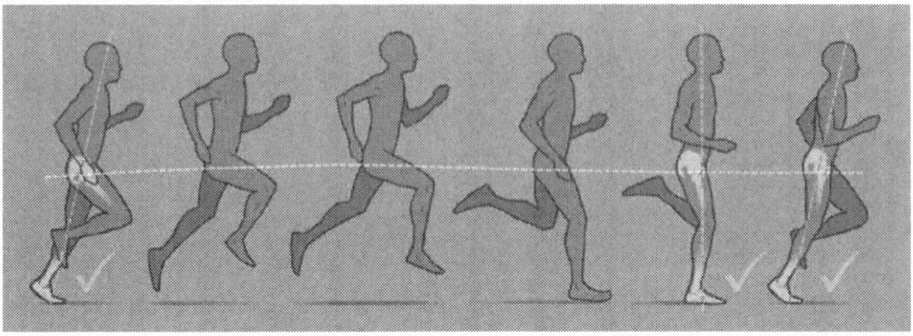

Illustration 18: *When running with good technique, the whole body leaves the ground. Note that this illustration is based on a runner travelling at 20 kilometres per hour, which causes the heel to spring up closer to the hips than at lower speeds.*

The faster you are travelling, the faster your foot will be pulled off the ground and the higher it will go. Your foot follows your hips, your knee rises up and forwards and, as your knee stops, your foot will fly further ahead before dropping under you.

Don't control your landings

Your body structure and the laws of physics will do it all for you. In other words, let things happen and be mindful not to 'drive' your knee forwards or consciously lift or try to place your feet. This is our eighth OYF Rule.

The second part of the take-off is the flight phase, which is the time between leaving the ground and your landing. There is a close relationship between this time in the air and your stride length. The height you reach from your take-off, and your speed determine your stride length.

Good runners spend an extended time in flight, and this is what gives them a long stride length. Accordingly, to increase your stride length, you should increase the time you stay airborne, not stretch out with your legs.

> ### OYF Rule #8: Don't try to control your feet
>
> A good runner's feet will rise off the ground—but are not lifted—and land in a particular way—but not forced. Similarly, your feet should rise naturally and there should be an almost instant whole-foot landing that is observed and felt, but not controlled. This will happen when you land balanced.
>
> Specifically:
> - Don't try to place your feet on the ground.
> - Don't lift your feet.
> - Don't try to land on any part of your foot: inside, outside, toes or heel.
> - Don't extend your stride length by reaching forwards with your feet.
> - Don't try to reduce your over-stride by doing faster, shorter steps.

3.3 Accelerating

When you start your run, you will be accelerating. You will need to tilt your body forwards and push forwards off your forefoot. The more you tilt, the more effort you need to put in, as tilting and pushing are interdependent.

When you are running at constant speed and want to increase speed, you use the same method to accelerate. However, it is usually better to concentrate on the power of your take-off and allow your body to tilt forwards naturally. We mention this here because some people think about leaning forwards too much and they end up bending over at the waist. This results in them swinging their leg forwards, causing them to over-stride.

Good examples of natural acceleration can be found by looking at kangaroos and how they use their powerful legs to bound forwards to extend their stride length, or how a unicyclist tilts forwards and pushes harder on their pedals to increase speed. Also, if you watch a 100-metre race, you will see how sprinters take off angled well forwards as they quickly accelerate down the track (see *Illustration 19*). Then, as they approach their maximum speed, they become more upright. Finally, when they have crossed the finish line they lean back so that their feet land in front of them to slow down.

Sprinters have to go from standing to maximum speed in the shortest possible time. They therefore have a very high cadence (the number of landings per minute) to spread the load. In contrast, distance runners will generally accelerate more gradually. Their cadence will only slightly increase as they increase speed.

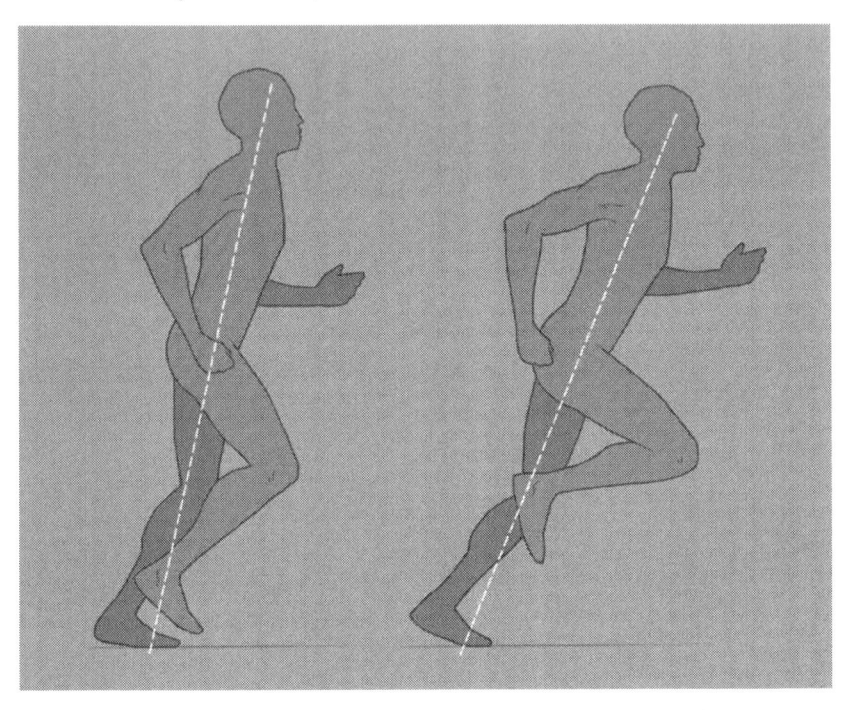

Illustration 19: To accelerate, take off in a more forwards direction. This requires a stronger take-off. If your acceleration is rapid, you will naturally increase your cadence to spread the load.

CHAPTER 4
INTRODUCING KEITH'S LESSONS

Keith Bateman

Before moving onto my lessons, let me remind you of the main aims of the book: to teach you how to run more efficiently (and hence faster) and to run injury free. To do this, you will need to change your current training, to commit to OYF Running and follow the exercises in both my lessons and *Heidi's Strengthening Program* (Chapter 11).

> *This will mean removing yourself from the racing scene so that you can rebuild your technique and your strength in the right areas.*

In Chapter 3, the running action was broken down into three phases: landing, take-off and accelerating. In the lessons that follow (Chapters 5 to 10), I show you how to put theory into practice and help you fix any problems you might have in attaining the ideal running action.

The techniques learnt in the early lessons are incorporated in the later lessons, and so the chapters and exercises should be done in sequence. After you have been through all the lessons once, you can practice any exercise in any order. My lessons are set up so that you can teach yourself in conjunction with the online videos and forum, which are accessible from our website, olderyetfaster.com.

In the first lesson (Chapter 5, *Lesson One: Landing*), I teach you how to land correctly. You might think that it would be more logical to start with your initial take-off, but landings are more important for two very good reasons:

- The feel of your whole foot contacting the ground provides you with excellent feedback to assess your running action, allowing you to constantly adjust balance.
- If you don't get the landing right, the whole running cycle will be compromised.

My landing exercises in the first lesson will allow you to practise landings in isolation from the rest of the running cycle. Once you know what the landing should feel like, then you can move on to take-offs.

In the second lesson (Chapter 6, *Lesson Two: Take-off*), I show you how to start off without over-striding.

The third lesson (Chapter 7, *Lesson Three: Accelerating*), covers acceleration.

By this point you will have learnt how to run with good technique throughout each part of the running action.

Lesson Four: Keith's Game Changer (Chapter 8) is where all components of the running action come together. In this lesson, you can expect to find your balance point, get your hamstrings (the long muscles at the back of the thighs) and glutes working, and give yourself that feeling of effortless running! It is also where you will get down to the real work and establish a platform for significant progress.

In the fifth lesson (Chapter 9, *Lesson Five: Going for a run*), I show you how to start off your runs. In this lesson, I give you a routine and some simple exercises to ensure you maintain good form in your warm-up. I then provide some guidance as to what to expect during your run. In the last part of the lesson, I also teach you how to handle hills.

Finally, in the last lesson (Chapter 10, *Lesson Six: Maintaining good form*), I show you ways to monitor and correct your running action. You will need this constant feedback to correct any bad habits you might fall into.

However, given that your existing running style has made you weak in several areas, you'll also need to build the necessary strength in your feet and legs while you follow the lessons. Therefore, *Heidi's Strengthening Program* (Chapter 11) should be done in parallel with Keith's Lessons, as she shows you how to build strength.

Then, in *Managing your transition* (Chapter 12), we show you how to manage your transition, and in *Heidi's rehabilitation exercises* (Chapter 13), we help you recover from injury.

All these chapters are part of the OYF Running experience and will give you the tools you need to achieve your best running action.

Technique change cannot be achieved overnight. It will take around six months of frequent, short sessions of steady running before you are strong enough to increase your workload. It will probably be another six months of gradually increased training before you are ready to think about racing.

There are also other factors that you need to take into consideration. When transitioning, you don't just have to keep working on your technique and cut back on the number of kilometres you run. You will also need to assess your footwear (see Chapter 14, *Shoes—what you need to know*). It's important that you do not undermine the benefits of all your hard work by continuing to wear chunky shoes. We recommend you upgrade to thin, flat, flexible shoes and add some barefoot running to your training. Remember that you should feel a whole-foot contact with the ground; the only way to do this is with the correct shoes. My lessons are best done barefoot on grass.

For more details about Keith's Lessons from a coach's point of view, see Appendix A, where I explain how to introduce OYF Running into your own coaching sessions.

CHAPTER 5
LESSON ONE: LANDING

Keith Bateman

Landing is the first of three lessons that I have designed to give you a new approach to your running. The techniques you will learn here are best practised every time you start off your runs, so you can refine them. In this first lesson, I teach you how to land with your foot in full contact with the ground and with your feet, hips and head all vertically aligned.

A balanced landing is key to learning how to run well and is the principle that underpins all of the lessons. To help you to achieve this, I get you to do three exercises: experimenting with foot contact, whole-foot landing and rebound, and finding the elasticity in your legs. You need to be able to do each of these exercises before moving on to the next one.

In EXERCISE 5.1, I get you to try and feel your whole-foot contact on the ground as you bounce up and down on the spot.

Then, in EXERCISE 5.2, I show you how to rebalance so that when you land you are using your whole foot for support. You will notice how this causes a vertical alignment of your whole body. The two actions are interrelated and together they will allow you to get all the benefits that flow from a balanced landing, such as reducing your braking, leaving the ground with less effort, and running faster.

Finally, in EXERCISE 5.3, I ask you to vary the tempo and height of your bounce by tightening and loosening your legs and feet muscles. By experimenting in this way, you will find out how to get off the ground with the least effort.

The breakthrough achievement of this lesson is when you become fully aware of your foot being in contact with the ground during your run, and can use this feedback to monitor and adjust your running action.

Before we start the landing exercises, bear in mind that the landing will feel more solid in these stationary exercises than in actual running. Also, the bouncing movement that I introduce you to will feel a bit awkward, but is necessary for you to experience the spring effect off the ground.

In order to land correctly, you need to feel what is happening when your foot comes into contact with the ground. This stationary exercise will give you the feedback you need by allowing you to experiment.

> EXERCISE 5.1: Experimenting with Foot Contact
>
> - Stand still and then bounce up and down on the spot on both feet.
>
>   Do you feel that you are landing on your toes? This is what most people do. I will show you how to change to a whole-foot landing in the next exercise.
>
> - Now, instead of landing on your toes, lean back slightly so you feel the landing on your heel bones. Be careful, as you will land with a thud! Do it very gently, and not on a hard surface.
>
>   Now you can understand how a small deviation from a vertically-aligned landing has a big effect on the way you land.

Now let's build towards a vertically-aligned, whole-foot landing.

> EXERCISE 5.2: Whole-foot Landing and Rebound
>
> - Start by bouncing up and down on both feet as in the first exercise, and gently rock backwards and forwards on the spot.
>
>   You will feel the pressure changing from the balls of your feet to your heels and back again.
>
> - Reduce this rocking motion until you find the point where your heel and forefoot land at the same time.
>
>   Your landings should feel a bit heavy at this stage, but don't worry; you won't feel this when you start running.

This whole-foot, vertically-aligned landing is what gives you maximum spring off the ground. This landing is what I am going to ask you to feel for later on, when you are running at constant speed.

It is important that you are able to achieve a whole-foot landing and a good rebound. You should get this exercise right before moving on to other exercises, as it will be fundamental to your running. See *Illustration 20*. This is our ninth OYF Rule.

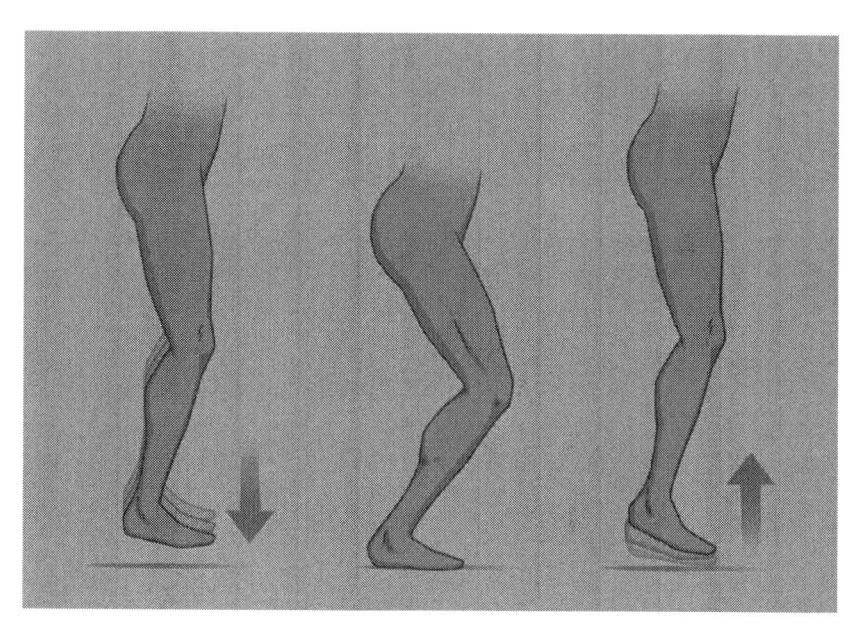

Illustration 20: *Whole-foot Landing and Rebound exercise. Land whole-foot (left, middle) and bounce off (right) the whole foot. Don't be too stiff or too soft. Feel the spring!*

OYF Rule #9: Aim for balanced whole-foot landings

A whole-foot landing is an important step in getting a balanced landing, as it gives you good feedback on your technique. You should feel even pressure between your forefoot and your heel. Bring your awareness to this contact of your foot on the ground until you have managed to correct your technique.

> At low speed, your heel will land firmly on the ground; you will feel a harsh, jarring sensation (think of a kangaroo hopping slowly). Once you speed up to about 6 minutes per kilometre, your landings will be much softer. You will eventually find the speed where it is even more efficient and you get a 'floating' feeling. For us, this starts at about 5 minutes per kilometre. Running starts to feel almost effortless as we approach 4 minutes per kilometre.
>
> In every run you will be a little off-balance at times—even the best runners won't manage a perfect landing every time. You might feel the ball of your foot or your heel touch a little too firmly; but, on average, you should feel your whole foot giving you complete support. However, do not make the mistake of 'placing' your foot on the ground or you will over-stride.

The height of your bounce is determined by the tightness or looseness of the muscles in your feet and legs. In the next exercise, I want you to vary this elasticity and hence change the strength and cadence of your bounce.

You will need to know how to adjust the flexibility in your legs on landing to correct your form when you run. This exercise is also done on the spot.

> EXERCISE 5.3: Elasticity in Your Legs
>
> - Bounce up and down on both feet as in the previous exercise.
> - As you bounce, let your legs slacken a bit so your tempo gradually slows.
>
>   You will find that you lose your spring and you will start feeling some stress in your quads. This is similar to the feeling you will get when the quads are stressed when you are over-striding during running (see *Illustration 21*).
>
> - Stiffen your legs again to regain your elastic bounce.
>
>   This is also something you can try while running.

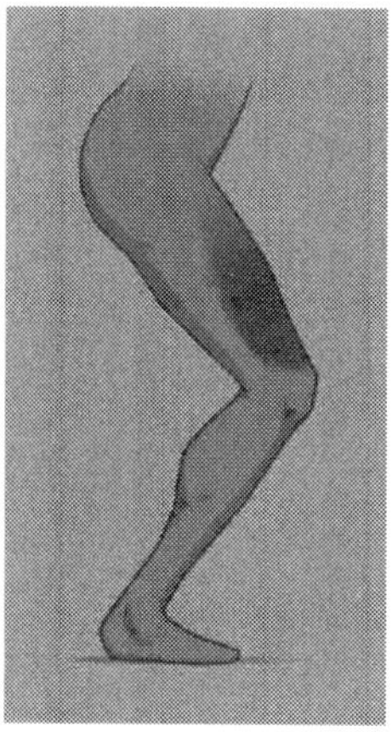

Illustration 21: Elasticity in Your Legs exercise. Slowing the tempo stresses the quads (dark area), in a similar way to over-striding.

Summary

In this lesson, I have taken you through three stationary exercises. The first two are the most important, as they show you how to establish a whole-foot, vertically-aligned landing. It is essential that you can do this consistently before moving on to the next two chapters: *Take-off* and *Accelerating*. In the third stationary exercise, I showed you that when you slow the tempo of your bounce you start to feel the stress on your quads, which is the same effect that you get when you over-stride. This idea of changing your leg tension is also presented as an advanced exercise in Chapter 10, *Lesson Six: Maintaining good form,* as it will help to correct your landings and find your balance point again.

CHAPTER 6
LESSON TWO: TAKE-OFF

Keith Bateman

In this lesson, I continue to get you to bounce, but this time in different directions so that you become familiar with a whole-body tilt, which will be used to accelerate. Then, using the bounce, you will start running. By combining this full-body tilt with standing tall, you will be starting off in good form.

6.1 Before you start

Each time you leave the ground, you are lifting a weight; so, just like a weightlifter, you need to have your whole body aligned to use your strength effectively. There should be a straight line through your ground-contact point, your hips and your head when you take off, and also when you land (see *Illustration 22*). If you focus on staying tall, you will normally achieve this without trying.

As mentioned, a big mistake that runners make when starting their run is to *walk* and not get off the ground. In this exercise, I show you how to overcome this error by bouncing up and down and then moving off with a full-body tilt. This tilt should be from the ankles and not from the waist.

Make sure when you are starting off, and when you are accelerating during your runs, that you keep these two things in mind: standing tall and tilting from the ankles.

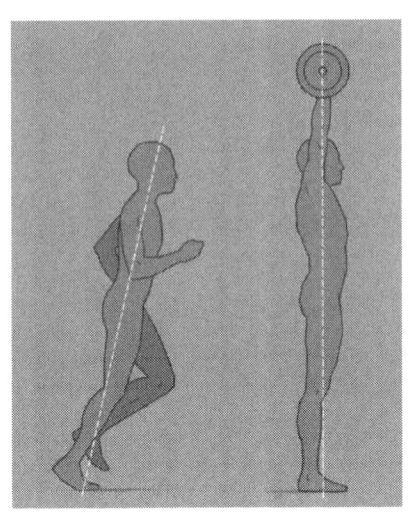

Illustration 22: Standing tall as you leave the ground is the strongest position to be in, just like a weightlifter pushing upwards. There should be a straight line through your ground-contact point, your hips and your head when you take off, and also when you land. Note that in a good take-off the 'free' foot is also aligned with the grounded foot, the hips and the head.

6.2 Using the bounce

EXERCISE 6.1: Bouncing and Tilting in Different Directions

- Stand tall and bounce up and down on both feet.
- Tilt your whole body *slightly* in the direction you want to go. You will naturally take off in that direction.

    Don't arch your back or bend from the waist. Make sure you are tilting from your ankle joint: your whole body should tilt, not just your upper body.

- Repeat this in all directions (see *Illustration 23*).

Note: Many of my clients find that the best to way achieve a full-body tilt is by moving their *hips sideways* first, then backwards, then forwards.

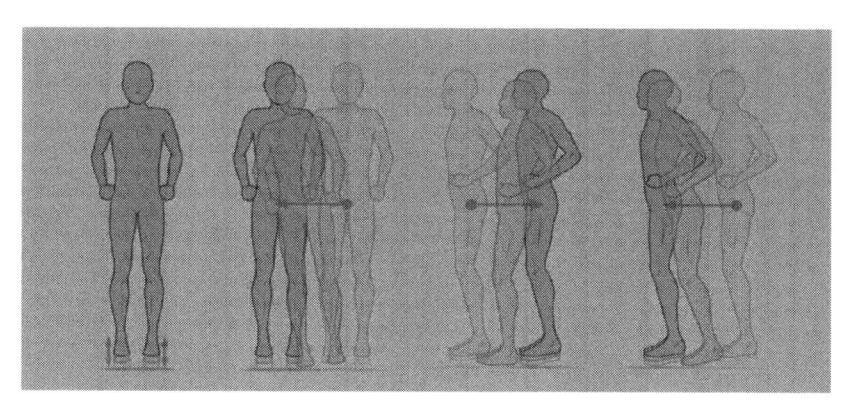

Illustration 23: *Bouncing and Tilting in Different Directions exercise. Bouncing on both feet (left) and then doing a whole-body tilt sideways (middle left), backwards (middle right), and forwards (right).*

> EXERCISE 6.2: Bouncing on Alternate Feet
>
> In this exercise, you bounce on the spot. However, this time you will be hopping from one foot to the other while keeping your shoulders horizontal, in preparation for starting to run.
>
> - Stand tall and bounce up and down on both feet.
>
> - While bouncing on both feet, move most of your weight onto one foot, keeping the toes of your other foot brushing the ground as you land.
>
> If your feet land exactly where they did when landing on both feet, you will have maintained your upright, aligned stance while on one foot. Note that on each landing, your heel will make *firm* contact with the ground.
>
> - Bounce on that foot for three bounces and then change to your other foot; just drop your foot each time you want to change feet. Keep your shoulders relaxed.
>
> - While still bouncing on one foot at a time, reduce the number of bounces on each foot until you are alternating: one bounce on each foot.
>
> Feel the bounce but also be relaxed with some flex in the legs: no shoulder rocking or 'Irish dancing' with stiff legs, and don't consciously lift your feet. When you can do this in a smooth and relaxed manner, you are ready to run.

6.3 Moving off in good form

It is now a simple procedure to start running by using the whole-body tilt, combined with your bouncy running on the spot. Remember to stay tall as you start, and as you continue in your run.

> EXERCISE 6.3: Bouncing on Alternate Feet and Tilting to Start Your Run
>
> - Repeat the previous exercise so that you are comfortably running on the spot.
> - Tilt your whole body lightly from your ankles (overbalance).
>
>   You will instinctively adjust your balance by taking off a little stronger. Tilting and pushing like this ensures that your feet naturally rise from the ground and drop perfectly under your hips.
>
> - Start off *very* slowly and allow your speed to build naturally.
>
>   You should continue to feel a solid, whole-foot landing as you did while stationary. Your landings will become lighter as your speed increases.
>
>   Do not stiffen your legs or lift your feet.
>
> - Emphasise the bounce-and-tilt action by bouncing and tilting backwards, and forwards a few times before moving gently into your run.
>
>   This will help prevent you from 'walking' your feet forwards.

6.4 Single-leg start

I sometimes use the single-leg start as an alternative method of starting off during running sessions with clients.

By restricting yourself to a hopping action, you cannot over-stride by walking forwards with the other leg. This exercise will get you used to 'tilting' and 'pushing' to start off. You will also feel the rebound when you manage to land balanced. Do this exercise gently with minimum effort and maximum balance. For best results, do it barefoot on grass.

> **EXERCISE 6.4: Single-leg Start**
>
> - Start off by standing on one leg. See *Illustration 24*.
> - Hop on one foot and gently tilt forwards to start moving.
>
>   Your foot should land firmly and flat. There should be no scuffing and there is no need to work hard when you get this right.
>
> - Build up momentum very gradually.
> - Do a few bounces on this first foot, landing as balanced as possible.
> - Then, stop and try this exercise on the other foot.
>
> When you can do these single-leg starts smoothly on each foot, you are ready to start swapping feet while moving.
>
> - While moving very slowly, do three bounces forwards on one foot.
> - Then, drop on to the other foot for the same number of bounces.
> - Keep swapping feet, gradually reducing the number of bounces on each foot until you are doing a very slow jog.
>
>   Get used to bouncing and allowing your foot to drop. Remain upright, with your head up. Use balanced whole-foot landings all the time and remember not to step forwards when you change feet.
>
> - Slowly build up speed by taking off with very slightly more power rather than increasing the cadence.

This exercise works well in combination with the *Beach check* (see Section 10.2, *Other checks and exercises to refine your form*).

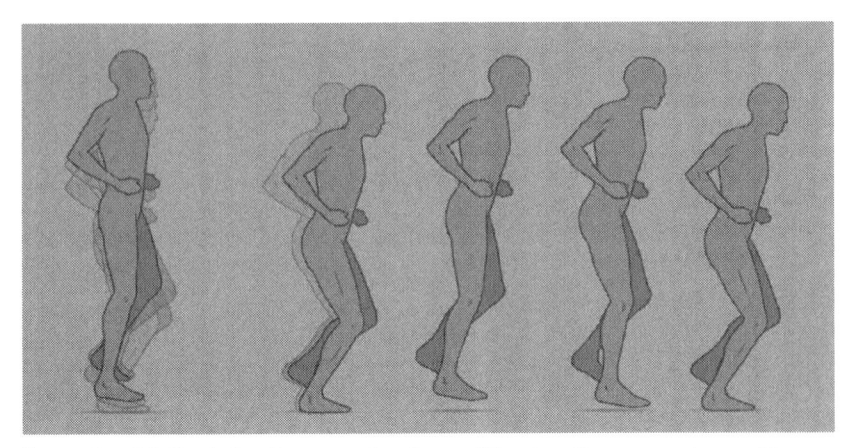

Illustration 24: Single-leg Start exercise. Start off by standing on one leg and bounce and tilt to accelerate. Your foot will follow and then drop under your hips. Make sure that you land your heel.

6.5 Summary

In this lesson, I showed you how to start off in the best possible way. I began by describing two things that you need to get right before you can do this: standing tall and tilting from the ankles. To get the idea of moving off with this full-body tilt, I got you to bounce in different directions. Then, I got you to bounce on alternate feet to start off your run in good form.

In the next lesson (Chapter 7, *Lesson Three: Accelerating*), I show you how the same principles apply to changing speed while you are already running. Please keep in mind the following notes:

- It is not the tilt that moves you forwards, but the strength of the push off the ground. The tilt causes you to overbalance and it forces you to push off more powerfully.
- While you are running, you only tilt to change speed. Your normal running position is very close to upright and relaxed, the same as when walking or standing.

CHAPTER 7
LESSON THREE: ACCELERATING

Keith Bateman

In the accelerating lesson, I complete the rebuilding of your running action by showing you how to accelerate by extending your stride length without over-striding.

A lot of people come to me with the misconception that all they need to do to accelerate is to increase their cadence. I tell them that if they do this they will only end up in a fast walk, rather than an efficient run.

When you are accelerating properly, many things change at the same time. However, there are three simple methods, which will not only give you a longer stride length but will allow you to run at your natural cadence. Luckily, all three methods affect each other and give the same results, meaning that you can use whichever method works best for you.

7.1 Accelerating by taking off more strongly

For the first method (main method), all you have to do is incorporate the whole-foot landing and full-body tilt that you have just learnt and add a bit more power to your take-off (see *Illustration* 25).

The easiest way to accelerate is to get higher off the ground. As with both other methods below, this will result in a longer stride length. Having established a whole-foot landing, simply tell yourself to take off with more power.

EXERCISE 7.1: Accelerating by Taking Off More Strongly

- Run at a constant speed and feel upright and balanced.

  Make sure you establish a whole-foot landing.

- Then, try to get very slightly higher off the ground by bending down a little to get an extra push off the ground (an extremely subtle action).

  This means that your foot will be on the ground slightly longer. As a result, your hips will travel farther ahead of your foot before you can leave the ground. Therefore, you will take off tilted slightly more forwards as well as slightly stronger (see OYF Rule #7).

  This will result in a longer stride length and you will accelerate.

  You will be surprised that with only a little more effort you will suddenly get a big increase in speed. You only need to tilt and push hard for a rapid acceleration. Practice your acceleration with a subtle change in effort, otherwise you might find that you go up too much and not forwards enough. If you keep feeling for a firm whole-foot landing, it should work very well.

Try the same acceleration on downhill slopes.

You can also feel this flying effect quite dramatically by jogging very slowly downhill (bounce your hips away from the ground rather than lifting your feet) and experiment by taking off a little higher, then lower, to change your speed. On the hill, the effect is magnified.

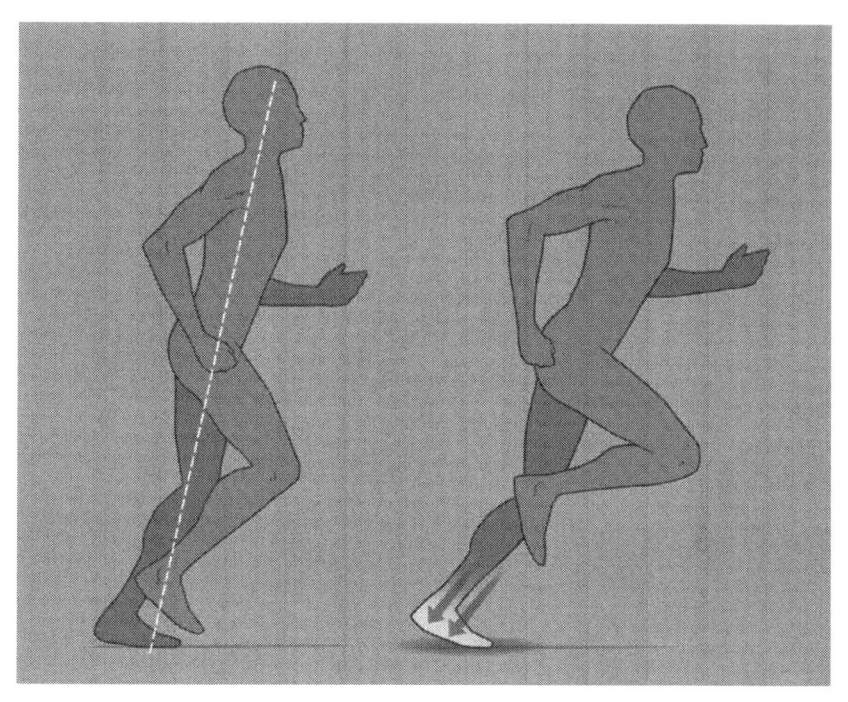

Illustration 25: Acceleration by Taking Off More Strongly exercise. Increasing your take-off power by trying to go up will result in a longer stride and more speed.

7.2 Accelerating by tilting more

For the second method, concentrate on taking off with a more forwards tilt. This will force you to put in a greater effort to get off the ground (see *Illustration* 26). However, you need to be careful not to overdo this tilt.

> EXERCISE 7.2: Accelerating by Tilting More
>
> - Run at a constant speed and feel upright and balanced.
> - Tilt forwards from the ankles, making sure this is a very subtle tilt.
>
> Increasing your forwards tilt will induce a stronger take-off, giving a longer stride and more speed.
>
> This should make you accelerate.

> However, if you overbalance too much, you will be left with no option but to over-stride by putting your foot on the ground in front of you.
>
> - After you have accelerated, tilt your body slightly back to upright, to continue at the new speed.
> - Repeat this acceleration a few times.

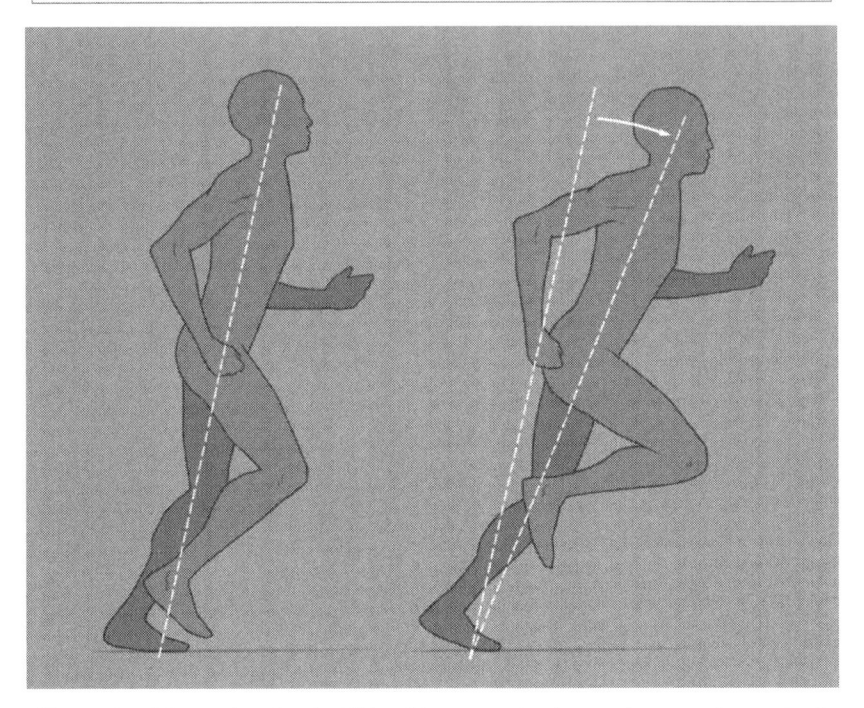

Illustration 26: Acceleration by Tilting More exercise. Increasing your forwards tilt (white arrow) will induce a stronger take-off, giving a longer stride and more speed.

The important characteristic shown in *Illustration 26* is that the whole body is tilted forwards. As mentioned earlier, sometimes when my clients first try this method they have a tendency to over-stride by bending from the waist and extending their leg to regain their balance. Tilting gently should be all you have to do to avoid this problem. But, if you find that you continue to have a problem, then try one of the other methods.

This method can also be used to 'reset' your form when you get tired. See also *The acceleration ladder* in Chapter 10, *Lesson Six: Maintaining good form*.

7.3 Accelerating by raising the back foot

You might have already noticed that, when you are running faster, your back foot rises higher off the ground. The third method uses raising your back foot to accelerate.

> EXERCISE 7.3: Accelerating by Raising the Back Foot
>
> - Run at a constant speed and feel upright and balanced.
>
> - Raise your back foot a few millimetres higher off the ground.
>
>   If you stand tall, a very small change in your foot height will have a big effect on your speed. With this in mind, just focus on raising your heel higher than it naturally goes and you will tilt forwards a little more and accelerate.
>
> - After you have accelerated, lower your foot again to continue at the new speed.
>
> - Repeat this acceleration a few times.
>
>   Remember to stay tall and effect only a slight rise. When you want to slow down, just slightly reduce the height of your heel.

Illustration 27 depicts the actions of accelerating and decelerating. The left figure shows running and then speeding up, and the right figure shows running and then slowing down.

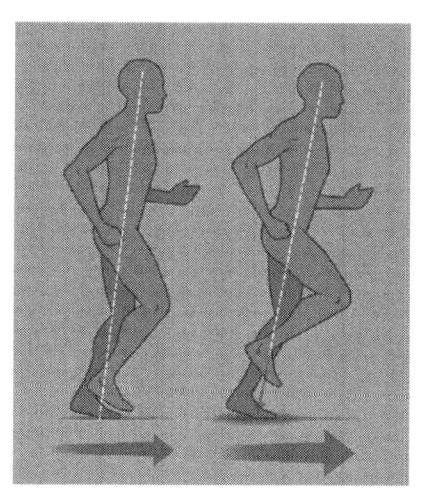

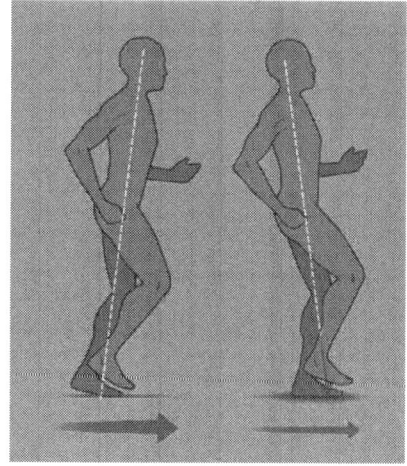

Illustration 27: Accelerating, showing degree of tilt (white) and amount of ground pressure (down-arrows). Left. Running and speeding up, with whole-body tilt forwards for more speed. Right. Running and slowing down, with whole-body tilt backwards to reduce speed.

7.4 Summary

My methods of acceleration encourage you to focus on a particular aspect of your running action. In the first method (EXERCISE 7.1), the focus is on a stronger take-off. In the second method (EXERCISE 7.2), the focus is on tilting forwards a bit more. And in the third method (EXERCISE 7.3), the focus is on lifting your back foot a little higher. These three factors are all interconnected and changing any one of them will cause a change in the other two. Likewise, the same three factors can be used to cause a deceleration. For example, when you lower your back foot, you will tilt backwards and reduce the power of your take-off and decelerate (*Illustration 27*, right).

Two other important things that change when you change speed are your stride length and cadence. Fortunately, you don't have to consider these. All you need to do is choose one of my methods and, if you get it right, you will find that your cadence and stride length will naturally adjust as well.

CHAPTER 8
LESSON FOUR: KEITH'S GAME CHANGER

Keith Bateman

Now that you are well on your way to achieving good technique, it is time to show you how to find your balance point.

Keith's Game Changer will show you how to combine what you have learnt in the last three lessons to find your perfectly balanced landing. When you can maintain balanced landings, your running will become smoother, faster and feel almost effortless.

As we've been discussing, if you want to run efficiently, you will need to remain vertically aligned each time you land. In the first exercise of this lesson, you will do the opposite of an over-stride and lean too far forwards. Then, in the second exercise, you will experiment landing with your body tilted at different angles until you find your balance point.

8.1 Preparation

Remember that the main running error is leaning back and landing with your feet too far in front of your hips. When running with an over-stride, your feet move close to the ground, land firmly in front of the body and your cadence is relatively slow.

The first exercise will cause your feet to be high off the ground, they will land slightly *behind* your hips, and your cadence will be relatively high. This is an exaggerated body position, which is the exact opposite of an over-stride.

The aim of this exercise is to make you eliminate this over-stride from your running action.

EXERCISE 8.1: Butt Kicks with Exaggerated Forwards Tilt

This exercise will make you lean too far forwards in preparation for moving into a balanced landing when running in the next exercise. See *Illustration 28*.

- Stand tall.
- Do high-frequency butt kicks on the spot with your knees held back.

    Feel yourself balancing on the balls of your feet.

- Tilt your whole body slightly forwards (balancing on your toes), so that you gradually move forwards.

    Take care not to advance too quickly, as this will mean that you are pushing your knees forwards and creating an over-stride.

- Continue doing this for a metre or two to make sure your form is solid and that you are not 'walking' forwards—keep those knees back.

    The better you can do this exercise, the better the result.

- Practice a few times before moving on to the next exercise.

    Good runners do good butt kicks!

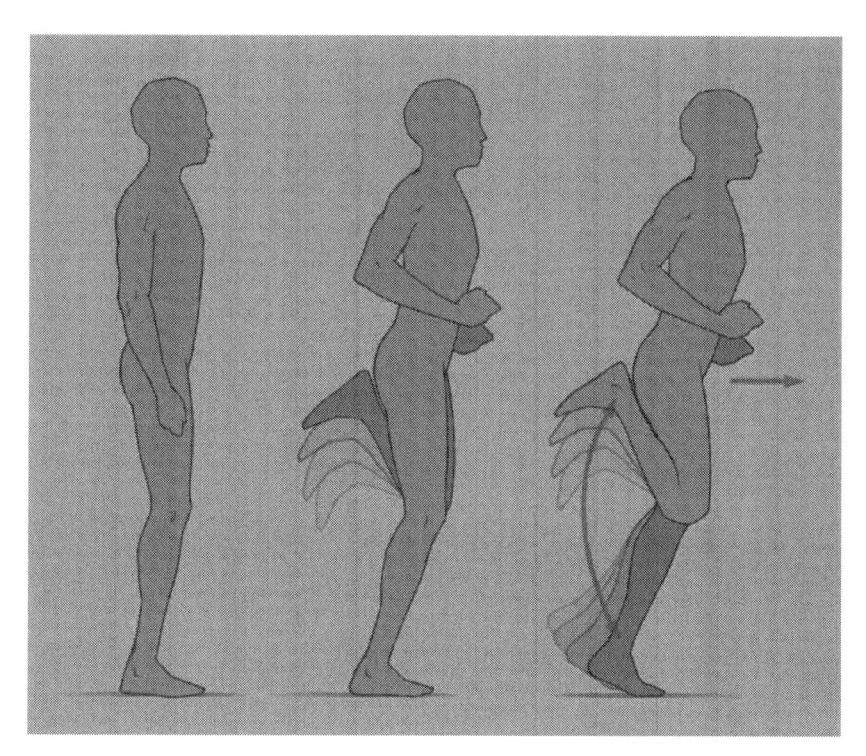

Illustration 28: Butt Kicks with Exaggerated Forwards Tilt exercise steps. Left. An upright stance. Middle. High-frequency butt kicks with your knees held back. Right. Balancing on your toes with very little forwards motion.

8.2 Finding your balance point

In the previous exercise, you started with a forwards tilt. In this exercise, you will gradually reduce this tilt until you find you are landing vertically aligned.

By gradually moving towards a more upright stance, you should find your balance point—somewhere between leaning forwards and leaning backwards.

When you do find this balance point, your running action will be instantly transformed, which is why I have called this lesson Keith's Game Changer.

EXERCISE 8.2: Butt Kicks Into a Fast Run

This exercise continues from the previous one.

- Start by doing the Butt Kicks with Exaggerated Forwards Tilt preparation exercise in which your feet land behind your hips.
- Overbalance a little more forwards—not too much—just enough to move a little faster.

  DO NOT allow your knees to go forwards yet!

- Get used to moving forwards in that fashion for a short distance, i.e. 3 or 4 metres.

  You will feel as if you are in a rather silly position. Doing this variation of butt kicks will feel like falling forwards as you kick your feet out behind you. But don't worry, all will come good as you perform the next part of this exercise.

Now your task is to gradually reduce the height that your feet kick up behind you, as you progress to a normal running action.

- Gradually reduce the kick as you increase speed, to the point where your feet are landing firmly under your hips.

  To do this, your body will have to become more upright and move towards the ideal running position. If you slowly reduce the kick as you speed up, you are sure to hit the 'sweet spot'.

  Remember to completely remove the 'kick' for this exercise to work. Also, you should no longer be trying to keep your knees back. See *Illustration 29* below.

- After a few attempts, increase your speed up to your maximum.

  This will give you a better chance of finding the 'sweet spot', as the height to which your feet are rising meshes smoothly with your speed.

  If you adjust your balance too quickly, you will go past the 'sweet spot' and your foot will start landing in front of your hips.

  When done right, you will transition from feeling the pressure on your forefoot to feeling your whole foot, as you have in the previous lessons. When you feel this, you will have reached your balance point.

If you repeat this exercise after all your warm-up and other exercises, it will continually reinforce good technique.

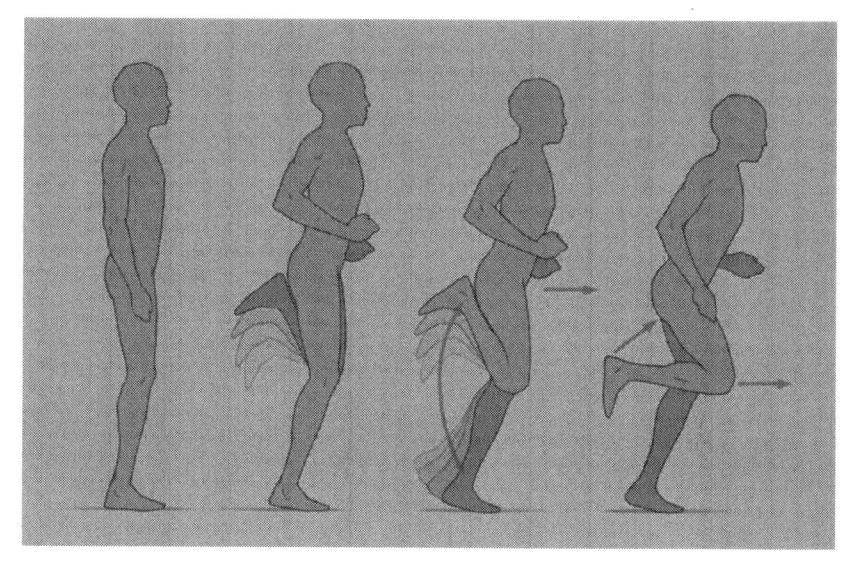

Illustration 29: Butt Kicks Into a Fast Run exercise. Left. An upright stance. Middle left. High-frequency butt kicks with your knees held back. Middle right. Butt kicks with your feet landing behind your hips. Right. Removing the butt kick by gradually reducing the kick as you increase speed to the point where your feet are landing firmly under your hips.

8.3 Summary

Keith's Game Changer is a lesson that I have developed to transform your running. You start by experimenting with your body tilted too far forwards. Then, you gradually reduce the tilt in an attempt to find your balance point. Once you have found this point, you will be landing vertically aligned and feel a whole-foot landing. You will also find that your running action feels smooth and effortless.

These two exercises are easy to practice, and well worth the effort, as you will find that what you achieve here is so rewarding. When you hit the right balance of cadence, power and angle, you will feel very smooth as you cruise at a constant speed. Regular practice will not only improve your landings but will also help you to build up weak glutes and hamstrings.

CHAPTER 9
LESSON FIVE: GOING FOR A RUN

Keith Bateman

Now that you have started to change your technique, your biggest challenge is to become comfortable with your new technique and not fall back into old habits. When I conduct my lessons, I am on the spot to give feedback to my clients. Therefore, I have included this chapter to provide you with the same guidance and reassurance that you need at this stage of your adjustment.

To help you keep your good technique, I have set out what you should be doing at each stage of your running sessions.

At the start of your runs, do the warm-up routine preparation exercises so that you begin with good form—reverting to your old style is common at the start of sessions.

Also, you will struggle to maintain good form if you start off too fast. Begin at a slow pace on a flat, smooth surface. Focus on getting a bounce from your landings and let your speed build up naturally.

Although most of your running should be on flat ground while you are perfecting your technique, you will certainly come across hills as you venture further afield. Therefore, at the end of this lesson, I show you how to run hills, as different factors come into play. You will need to vary your technique for both uphill and downhill.

9.1 Checking your form

Unless you are new to running, your old running movements will be etched in your brain. To begin the process of unlearning, you need to start off by doing the right things. The following three warm-up exercises will help you check your form at the beginning of your run.

> EXERCISE 9.1: Starting Off
>
> - Bounce on both feet to get vertically aligned.
>
>   See EXERCISE 5.2: Whole-foot Landing and Rebound.
>
> - Alternate your feet.
>
>   Make sure you are still bouncing rather than lifting your feet (see EXERCISE 6.2: Bouncing on Alternate Feet).
>
> - Practice tilting alternately backwards and forwards a few times.
>
>   This will encourage you to bounce and tilt rather than 'walk' your feet along the ground.
>
> - While still bouncing, tilt very gently forwards to start your run (see EXERCISE 6.3).

After running a few metres, use EXERCISE 9.2: Back-foot Check (see *Illustration* 30) and then, after another ten metres do EXERCISE 9.3: The 360-degree Spin (see *Illustration 31*) to make sure you have started correctly.

> EXERCISE 9.2: Back-foot Check
>
> - While running, look under your arm, back towards your heel, as in *Illustration 30*.
>
> - Move your head only enough to see your heel 'peeling' off the ground as your hips go ahead of your foot.
>
>   Remember, let your foot 'follow' you (OYF Rule #7), do not lift it (OYF Rule #8).
>
> This exercise prevents you from swinging or sweeping your legs forwards, as it forces you to tilt further forwards, cancelling out any backwards leaning. And because you will be watching your foot, it helps stop any foot-lifting. Don't run into anything!

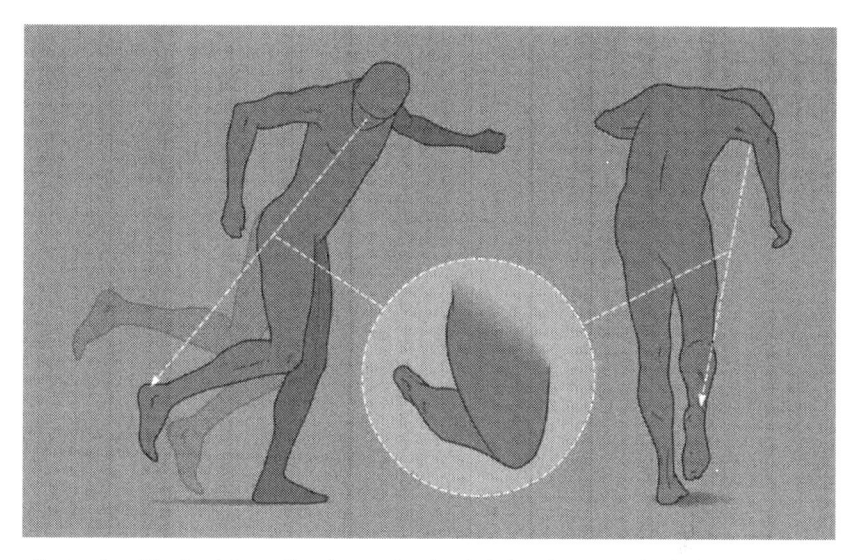

Illustration 30: Back-foot Check exercise. Look behind you to check that your back foot is moving the right way. If you have habitually been a heel-striker then this should get you balanced.

Once you have practised this exercise at the start of your runs you might find that just thinking about the action of your foot as it rises towards your hamstrings will help you achieve a more balanced landing. See Chapter 10, *Lesson Six: Maintaining good form*, for more re-balancing ideas.

EXERCISE 9.3: The 360-degree Spin

- While running slowly, spin 360 degrees without slowing down. See *Illustration 31*.

    Do not hesitate as you go into the spin.

- When you are coming out of the spin, continue running smoothly for at least 4 or 5 landings.

- Alternate clockwise spins with anticlockwise spins.

    Do not worry that you need to be on your toes while you are rotating.

    The important thing is to be balanced after the rotation.

If you succeed in rotating in a continuous motion, your body will be aligned both when landing and on take-off; and you will be running with good form.

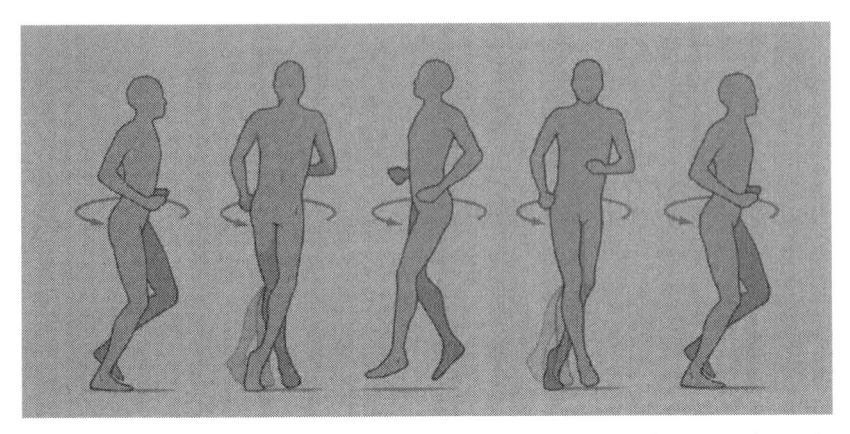

Illustration 31: The 360-degree Spin exercise. While running, make a seamless spin like a dancer or ice skater.

9.2 What should happen during your run

Every run should start with a 2 or 3 kilometre warm-up. If you are new to running, then your whole run could be called a warm-up, but as you add sufficient distance to your runs, there will be three distinct stages: a warm-up, the run itself, and the cool-down.

Warm-up

Always start your run with a warm-up using the following exercise. It incorporates the above starting routine and the two checks to start running correctly.

> EXERCISE 9.4: Warm-Up
>
> - Check your form by doing EXERCISE 9.1, EXERCISE 9.2 and EXERCISE 9.3.
>
> - Keep running very slowly and feel for a firm, whole-foot landing as evidence that you are landing close to vertically aligned.
>
>   At the start, your landings will be hard because there will be a lot of vertical motion and very little forwards motion.
>
> - Focus on staying tall and looking straight ahead. Go slow and relaxed.

> You will probably find that the most difficult thing to do is hold back from going too fast at the beginning of your run. As your muscles warm up, you will naturally bounce a little easier off the ground. This will increase your stride length and speed with no extra effort and you won't notice it happening until you get out of breath!

Your run

The run is a continuation of the warm-up. The runner does absolutely nothing different, but heart rate, speed, cadence, stride length, breathing, etc. all change as the muscles, tendons and ligaments become more efficient.

Below are some rough guidelines you can use to monitor your progress over the period of your transition. But don't start thinking about these measurements until *after* your run: your running should be about 'feel' and not formulas. The given measurements are only indicators and no one measurement on it's own should be focused on, or is valuable on it's own.

During your run, your landings will also become smoother as you speed up.

> **EXERCISE 9.5: Your Run**
>
> Your run is simply a continuation of your warm-up.
>
> - Continue your slow running, feeling for nothing more than your firm support from a whole-foot landing and the little rebound that gives you.
>
>   Your body movement should continue to be mostly up and down.
>
> - You need to do nothing else—just try to maintain balanced landings and allow your muscles to warm up.
>
> As your muscles warm up, your speed will naturally increase and your cadence will settle into your optimal range. When you are finally going faster, you may even feel that you are doing less! After two or three kilometres, you should have naturally speeded up and all you need to do is focus on the exercises of your choice from the next chapter, *Maintaining good form*.

> If you have taken measurements with a smart watch during your run, these are the results you are likely to see once you have finished your run:
>
> - The first kilometre, in 6 or 7 minutes, with a cadence of around 170 to 180 steps per minute.
>
> - The second kilometre, about 1 minute quicker than the first kilometre, with a slightly higher cadence.
>
> - The third kilometre, about 30 seconds quicker than the second, with a cadence of probably between 180 and 185 steps per minute.
>
> You should be fully warmed up after 3 kilometres and this is all you should do on your first run.

Cool-down

Remember to do a cool-down at the end of your run. In the early stages of your transition you might only need to walk home for a cool-down. When you are training harder and faster, do a few kilometres of easy jogging.

Building distance

If you are new to running, or you are using running as a way of starting to regain fitness, then you might initially manage only a few hundred metres before getting out of breath. This is not unusual. Once you can repeat the above two exercises three times a week, you will be able to build distance.

When you go for a run, you just need to keep all of Keith's Lessons in mind and let the good results flow naturally. Don't start out thinking that you need to run at a set speed or achieve a predetermined cadence. Many experts set these artificial targets, but this approach just moves the emphasis away from good technique and interferes with the natural process.

Thereafter, your running distances will depend on how your calf muscles are coping with the workload. This is described in more detail in Chapter 12, *Managing your transition*.

In the early days of your transition, you should stick to flat ground and constant-speed running, introducing some speedwork and hills once you are comfortably running 5 kilometres. However, some hill running will be unavoidable as you increase your range, so you might like to make yourself familiar with the techniques for running up and down hill by reading the following section now.

9.3 Running hills

You may think that running hills is not much different to running on the flat. You are right up to a point. Running on all surfaces involves the same components. However, just like running on a flat but uneven surface, running up and down hills involves additional factors. With this in mind, before you tackle substantial hills, I recommend that you establish good technique on consistent flat surfaces or slight inclines only.

When running up a hill, you will need to tilt forwards and push slightly harder to extend your stride length, as this has been reduced by the slope. If the hill is steeper, you will need to tilt even more and push even harder to maintain speed.

Conversely, when running down a gentle decline, you will need to tilt back and take off a little less strongly off the ground. On a steeper hill you will have to lean back further and start pushing against your direction of travel to maintain a constant speed. It is especially important when running downhill that these actions are smooth and gradual.

Note: If the angle of the down slope is just right, then you will actually take off vertically and this is the basis for the Downhill Sprints (EXERCISE 10.6) in Chapter 10, *Maintaining good form,* where the gentle slope will enable you to 'float' down the hill with no discernible braking.

Uphill

Once you are happy that you have achieved good technique when running on the flat, you can try uphill. When approaching a hill, you will need sufficient speed. If you start fast enough, you can concentrate on going *up* and allow your momentum to carry you forwards. Just like trying to ride a bike slowly up a hill, running up a hill slowly doesn't work:

at low speed it is easier to walk. So, hit the hills with confidence and speed and you will be less likely to lose your good form.

When running uphill (see *Illustration 32*), the ground rises towards you and this will cause you to naturally shorten your stride. Some things to keep in mind:

- You will need to take off more strongly to maintain your stride length and speed.
- You will probably find that, as you try to increase the power of your take-off, your cadence will increase automatically.
- You are unlikely to increase speed on the hill. Just try to keep your good form so that you do not slow down and make your run harder than it should be.
- Unless the hill is very slight, your heel may not touch the ground.
- Your foot must never land in front of you. In fact, try to feel for it landing behind you.
- You shouldn't lift your knees, as this will not help the rest of your body rise up the hill. Your knees will rise as your whole body rises as a unit.
- Simply stand tall and make sure your heel rises towards your hamstring. Think of this as a mental trick to find the right action, rather than a foot-lifting exercise.
- If running up hills feels relatively easy and you maintain a reasonable speed, then you have achieved the right balance.

When you start to feel tired, remember not to let your body sink lower or sit back by lifting your knees. A good tip to avoid falling into this crouched position is to stretch up and fall slightly into the hill as you move onto it.

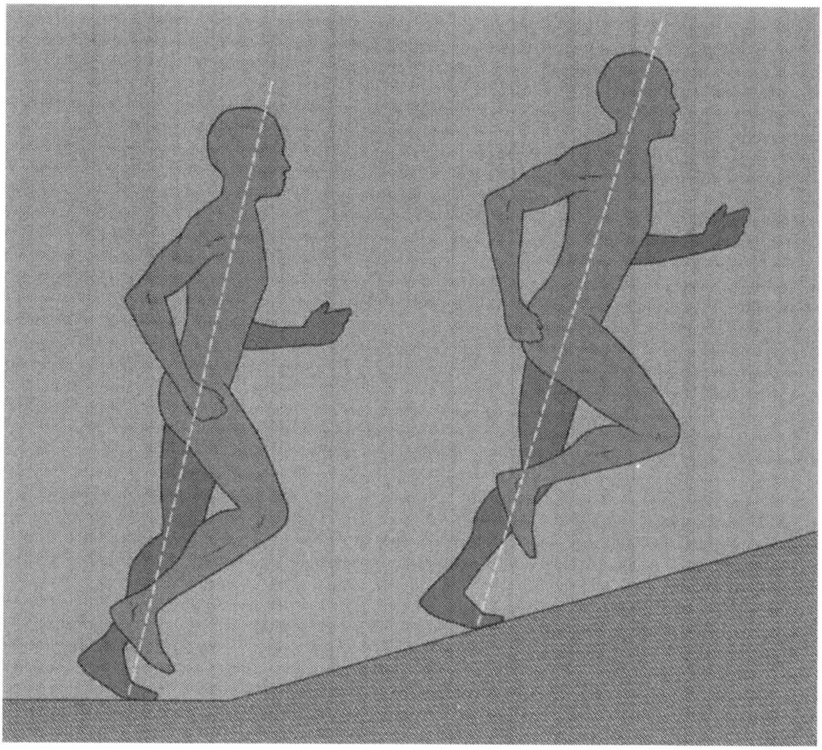

Illustration 32: Uphill running. Simply standing up and making sure your heel is moving towards your hamstrings is all that is needed as a cue for most people to start running uphill with good form.

Downhill

It is difficult to run smoothly downhill and it takes years of practice to get really good at it. You need to concentrate on every step to avoid getting out of control, and there is always the problem of over-stressing the quads and knees when you over-stride and have to brake too harshly.

When running downhill, you actually HAVE to over-stride a little to control your speed, but if you are adding this to an existing over-stride, the descent will become rough and unbalanced and can damage the body. Poor technique also makes it much more likely that you will slip and turn an ankle when running downhill, especially on wet or loose surfaces.

General tips on running downhill:
- As you are approaching the downhill slope, be aware that you might need to brake gently if it is a steep decline. On a short hill you can often let yourself go, but longer hills require more control by using less take-off power to minimise braking.
- It is best to practice on gentle declines and to work towards steeper declines, as you will not have to brake so hard and you will be able to focus more on your technique. The steeper the slope, the more you will need to make sure that your stride length and speed do not increase beyond what you are comfortable with.
- You will probably find that, as you decrease the power of your take-off to keep a constant speed, your cadence will decrease slightly. But there should be no dramatic change in your cadence from flat to downhill.

Technique tips on downhill running:
- Throughout the descent, remain tall and feel for a balanced whole-foot landing (the temptation is to reach out with the heel). Try to push your foot flat onto the hill to make sure you are not over-striding.
- Restrict the height your back foot rises. This will gradually tip your body backwards and cause your other foot to land a little further ahead of your hips to slow you down—but it will be controlled and it will keep you stable. This trick is also very useful when approaching the hill.
- Experiment with differing amounts of take-off power and leg speed to make your downhill run as smooth as possible.

9.4 Summary

Having just covered the essentials of changing your technique in the previous four lessons (Chapters 5 to 8), this lesson provides you with some of the support that you would get during my technique-change sessions. The point of this lesson is to encourage you to continue running well and to avoid falling back into bad habits.

I suggest that you get comfortable with your technique change on the flat or slight inclines before tackling steeper slopes. This is because other factors come into play for both uphill and downhill running.

CHAPTER 10
LESSON SIX: MAINTAINING GOOD FORM

Keith Bateman

Now that you are putting the lessons into practice, you will need to work hard at maintaining your good form.

In the first section of this chapter, I show you how to detect and correct any faults in your running technique by doing some simple exercises during your run. I would normally introduce these exercises to my clients in my sessions, and get them to try out a few until they find one that works best. You should do the same.

In the second section, I show you how to refine your technique using further running checks that require a specific environment. These checks are usually done separate to your run and will highlight deficiencies in your running action, such as over-striding and lack of balance.

10.1 Ways to check your form during your run

Start by selecting one of the exercises below and incorporate it into your run. As you are running, make the adjustment that the exercise requires. You should find that it improves your technique on the go.

The pendulum

The pendulum exercise has two parts and will help you find the balance point of your landing. Consider this an exercise of 'getting it wrong to get it right'. It shows you how, by accentuating the feel of being off-balance—both backwards and forwards—you can find the ideal middle point.

> EXERCISE 10.1: Preparation for the Pendulum (stationary)
>
> Do this preparation before you start moving, to get a feel for your balance point by rocking backwards and forwards on the spot.
>
> - Stand barefoot with your eyes closed.
> - Gently rock backwards to apply pressure to your heels.
> - Rock forwards onto your forefoot, and then onto your whole foot.
>
>   You will be moving like a pendulum, hence the name of this exercise.
>
> - Then, perfect this motion by adjusting the pressure on the ground, rather than by swaying your body.
>
>   You should now be able to make fine adjustments to your stance without swaying your body.

Now, start running and do the next part of the exercise.

> EXERCISE 10.2: The Pendulum (moving)
>
> This part of the pendulum exercise (shown in *Illustration 33*) takes you through three sequences (A, B, C) of backwards leaning, forwards leaning and then landing balanced.
>
> As you progress from A to B, and B to C, the angles at which you lean, become closer to the vertical in each sequence. Each sequence ends with a balanced, upright stance.
>
> - While running, tilt back so that you start landing with your feet well in front of you (yes, you will be over-striding!)—see *Illustration 33*, sequence A, left figure.
> - Do this for four to six landings.
>
>   You will slow down, but make sure you maintain some speed so you can perform the rest of the exercise well.
>
> - Then, tilt your whole body well forwards so that your toes land well behind you. You should start to accelerate again—see *Illustration 33*, sequence A, second figure.

- Ease into an upright position where you can feel your whole foot landing. Do this slowly so that you can maintain your speed—See *Illustration 33 B*, right figure.

  You are trying to find that 'effortless running' position between deceleration and acceleration.

- Keep running and repeating the above steps with progressively smaller amounts of tilt, until you feel the perfect balance point (*Illustration 33 B* for less tilting, then *C*, and so on).

After your first attempt at this exercise, you will only need to practice the final, more precise, part where changes in your balance are very slight, and you can feel these changes simply by pressure under your feet.

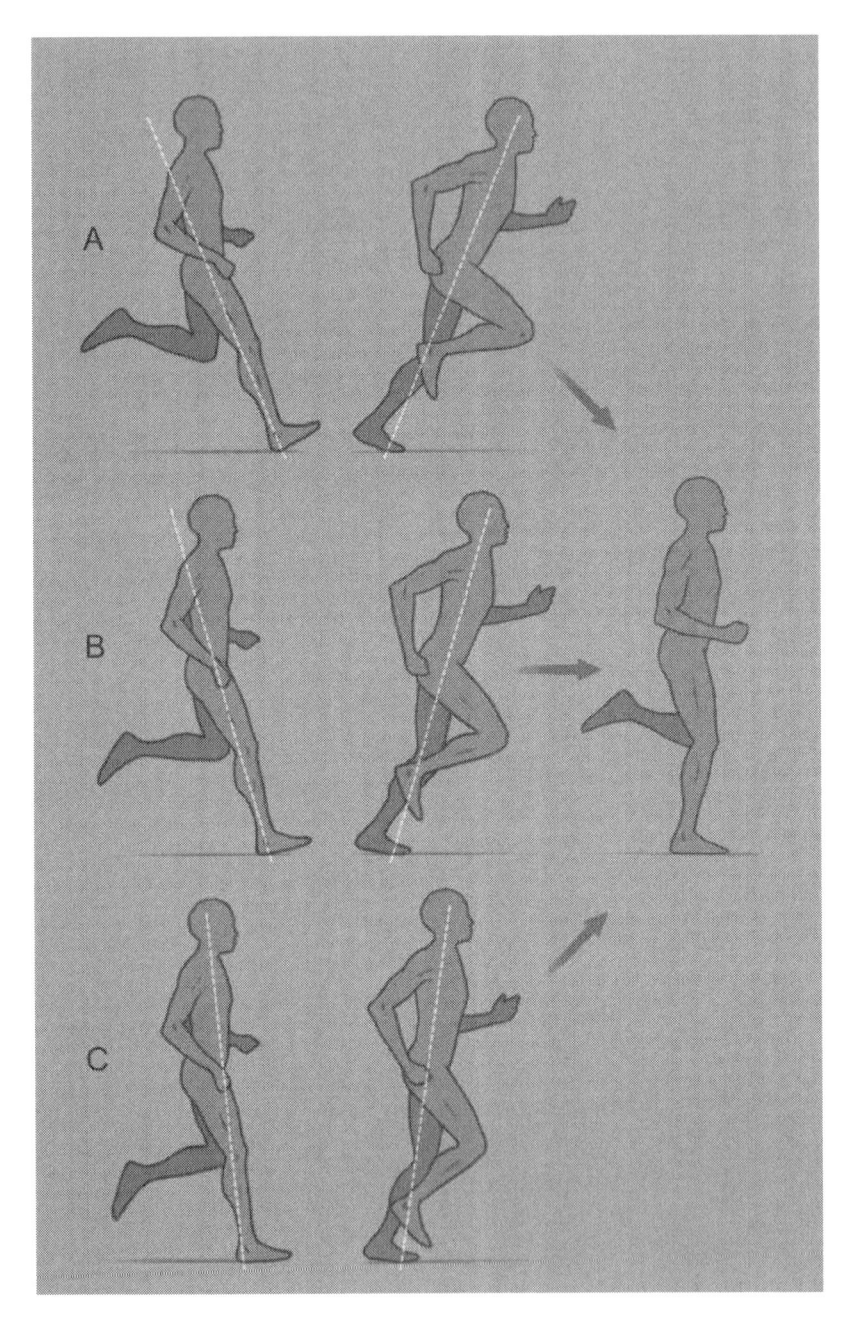

Illustration 33: *The Pendulum (moving) exercise. The three alignments during the pendulum exercise. Depicted are multiple sets of backwards tilt, forwards tilt, then upright. Begin with the most pronounced (A) tilt then reduce the tilt in each set (B) and (C).*

The acceleration ladder

This exercise is Heidi's favourite: 'I spent so much time leaning back, this exercise helped me position my torso over my hips'.

> EXERCISE 10.3: The Acceleration Ladder
>
> - While running at a steady pace, tilt gently forwards.
>
>   This will induce an acceleration.
>
> - Gently return to your vertical position, making sure to maintain your new faster speed.
>
>   What you have just done is the same as the acceleration (tilting forwards) part of the pendulum in EXERCISE 10.2.
>
> - Repeat this over and over, each time going to a higher constant speed (the next rung of the ladder) until you reach maximum speed.
>
>   You should feel the pressure towards the ball of your foot when accelerating, and then on your whole foot as it lands under you when running at constant speed.
>
> Make sure you are not bending over at the waist as you tilt forwards, or you will start over-striding by advancing your leg to balance your head and torso. If you think this is happening, then accelerate by taking off more strongly instead of tilting.

Back-foot adjustment

This exercise shows an alternative way of finding your balance point by raising and lowering your heels. Raising your heels should move your balance point forwards, and lowering them should move it backwards. A small movement of only a few millimetres is very effective.

> EXERCISE 10.4: Back-foot Adjustment
>
> - During your run, raise your heels too high for a few strides.
>
>   You should start accelerating, as you need to tilt forwards to balance your feet.
>
> - Lower your heels very low to the ground.
>
>   Your body will tilt back and you will slow down.

- Next, raise your heels again.
- Gently lower you heels until you feel balanced and are running at a constant speed.

This should be a very subtle movement.

Stand tall and reset

During running, when your muscles are fatigued, your hips will drop closer to the ground and your feet will land too far in front of you. This means you will be absorbing excess pressure on each landing. This affects your ability to spring off the ground. The best way to regain the spring in your step is by training yourself to stand tall at these times.

This simple adjustment is the best thing you can do to regain this spring. Your foot will automatically start landing more under your hips, aligning your body to take advantage of the elasticity in your legs. But take care not to stand up and lean back.

The following exercise shows three separate tricks to combine with standing tall. For all three, you should first stand tall and then make the adjustment shown. After you have tried them all, choose the one that works the best and incorporate that in your running.

EXERCISE 10.5: Stand Tall and Reset

This is a correction exercise for when you start to fatigue. Try each of the following three correction methods and choose the one that works best for you.

- 1. Tuck your pelvis under, so that you don't have a curve in your lower back.

  You will feel that rebound again.

- 2. Tilt forwards slightly from the ankles to ensure you do not sit back.

  This will bring your feet back just like an acceleration, but just enough to rebalance your landings.

- 3. Stand tall and aim your heel approximately towards the back of your knee to make sure you are not swinging your leg forwards—this is shown below in *Illustration 34*.

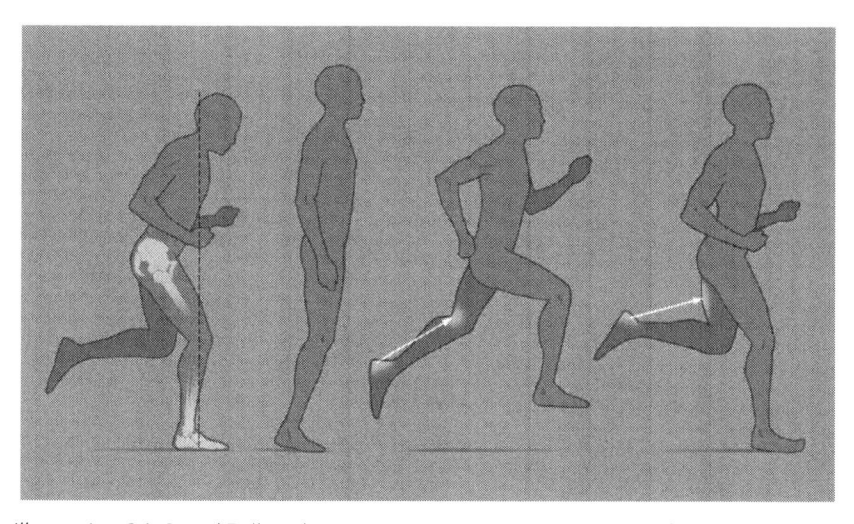

Illustration 34: Stand Tall and Reset exercise, correction method 3 for when you start to fatigue. While running, stand tall and then aim your heel at your hamstrings (think 'back of the knee' as a good approximation).

If you are tired and you regain a well-balanced landing from doing this exercise, you might feel your glutes working each landing. If you do, you are doing very well and are probably running very fast!

Adjusting your spring and take-off power

Two useful methods you can use while training to encourage good form and build strength are:

- Adjust the spring tension in your legs (make your legs slightly stiffer as you land, as you did in EXERCISE 5.3). This will make your feet land more under your hips and give you a little more lift off the ground. You should feel a slight acceleration when you try this, due to your body taking off higher from the ground.
- Slightly slow your cadence while keeping the same speed. This is an advanced method for when your speed is naturally exceeding 5 minutes per kilometre and your cadence is automatically above 185 steps per minute. It will get you used to a more powerful take-off. Clients who have tried this method in training for a few weeks have often seen a big improvement in their race times.

Making it wrong to make it right

Let's try some wrong movements now, and then correct them. This will show you how the wrong movements affect your performance.

While running:

- Rotate your shoulders, then stop the rotation.
- Lift your knees up, then stop lifting your knees up.
- Bend forwards at the waist (crouch down and feel your quads burn), then stand tall and aim your heel towards your hamstrings.
- Kick your feet up behind you, then stop kicking your feet up.

Can you feel the difference?

10.2 Other checks and exercises to refine your form

The previous exercises can be done on any run. Most of the checks below require a specific environment.

Dusty-track check

If you are over-striding, you will be braking on each landing and accelerating on each take-off.

On dusty ground, you might feel your shoe slip back as you take off, sometimes leaving a skid mark on the ground. This means you are pushing yourself forwards too hard to compensate for too much braking on landing. You can feel the same effect on any sand-covered, or slippery, hard surface.

If your over-stride is particularly bad, you might even slide forwards on landing too. Feel what's happening and listen for the 'chh, chh, chh' noise as your foot slips backwards or forwards along the ground.

To fix this, keep your foot dorsiflexed (point your toes towards your shin) as your foot leaves the ground. This will stop you 'driving' forwards or 'toe-running'.

Beach check

The better the runner, the less they need to push off their forefoot to maintain a constant speed. Therefore the best runners will leave a smooth, minimal imprint in the sand.

See *Illustration 15* in Section 3.2, *Take-off*, for samples of good and bad footprints in the sand. The less disturbance in the sand the better, as shown in the bottom footprint. You will only leave a smooth footprint when you are in perfect balance. Even when you are not on a beach, you can use this check to help you towards balanced landings by imagining you are landing in this way.

If you are digging out a lot of sand, once again, try keeping your ankle dorsiflexed as it leaves the ground. This will stop you pushing forwards (off your forefoot) and will likely move you into a more balanced landing position.

Water check

If you are running well, you can run straight through shallow water without the water affecting your technique. This is because your feet are only going forwards when they are above the water. Your feet rise towards your hips on their way out of the water, and on the way down they fall backwards in relation to your hips, entering the water with almost no forwards motion. If you are over-striding you will find that your feet catch the water as they swing forwards.

Start off running in shallower water then move deeper. Be careful not to adjust your technique by lifting your feet to keep them out of the water. If the water is deep enough to catch the toes of your back foot you have reached your depth limit. See *Illustration 35*—note the near-vertical plume of water after the foot leaves the water if your technique is good.

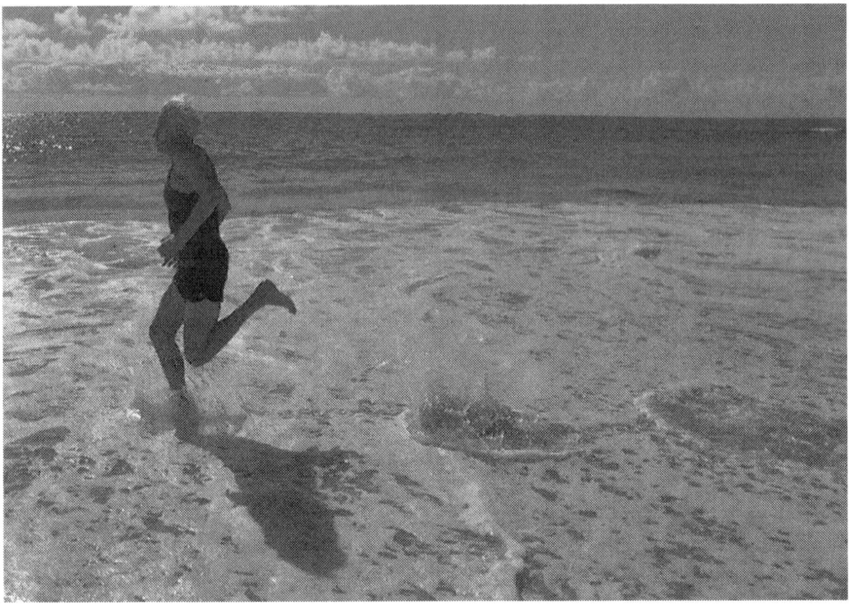

Illustration 35: Water check. This photo, taken just before the landing is completed, shows how the foot enters and leaves the water with minimum disturbance. The water from the splashes is near-vertical in response to the landings, which are also near-vertical. Photo by Stuart Greaves.

This trick also works in long grass. Try not to 'grass cut' with your feet. Listen for the noise and amend your technique so the noise stops (stand tall and ensure your heel moves towards your hamstrings without lifting it).

Run barefoot on a hard surface

Firstly, check your running surface to make sure it is free of obstacles (stones, sticks, glass and so on). A concrete pavement, tiled area or inside a sports hall is ideal.

Running on these smooth, solid surfaces is the best way to get a feel for a smooth and balanced landing, and to get great feedback so you can continually improve. This is because such surfaces will magnify any imperfections in your technique. I do this most days to maintain my form. You will find that 100 metres is enough at first.

Leaning back slightly is a common error, as it is natural to err on the side of caution when running barefoot on a hard and untried surface. This lean will result in you landing heel first, and you will hear the slap as the front part of your foot lands. Use one of the re-balancing exercises (such as EXERCISE 10.2: The Pendulum (moving), EXERCISE 10.3: The Acceleration Ladder, and EXERCISE 10.4: Back-foot Adjustment) to adjust your whole-body balance so you get a whole-foot landing. Do not adjust the angle at which your foot lands and do not place your foot on the ground or lift it. Let your feet fall naturally and, when you are well balanced, your landings will be good.

Downhill sprints

For this exercise, find a gentle slope to run down, where you don't have to worry about going too fast and needing to brake. The downward slope will give your foot more time to move under your hips and negate some of your natural braking.

> EXERCISE 10.6: Downhill Sprints
>
> At the top of the hill, do the warm-up routine in EXERCISE 9.1: *Starting Off*.
>
> - Stay tall and start running downhill.
> - Allow your speed to build gradually.
> - Feel for whole-foot contact with the ground on each landing.
> - Reach a speed where you are on the verge of going too fast but feeling balanced.
>
>   You should feel the 'float' that top runners feel when they land perfectly balanced.

Good and bad technique on the treadmill

These exercises use a treadmill. A treadmill not only gives a smooth, even surface under foot, but it also reduces external factors and enables you to focus on certain aspects of your running action.

In these exercises, you will be highlighting the difference between good and bad technique using three different ways of accelerating.

First, I get you to simulate two common errors of technique that runners fall into when trying to accelerate: accelerating by advancing your foot in an over-stride, and accelerating by unnecessarily increasing your cadence.

After you have seen how both of these acceleration techniques involve a lot of effort, I then get you to try accelerating by increasing the power of your take-off to spend more time in the air. Once you can do this, you will find that the latter technique is easier and by far the most efficient way to accelerate.

First, make sure the treadmill is not set on an incline.

> EXERCISE 10.7: Accelerating by Increasing Your Over-stride
>
> - Stand on the treadmill and start it at the lowest speed.
> - As the treadmill belt starts moving, start off at walking pace.
> - Gradually increase the speed of the treadmill and, as the belt speeds up, make longer strides by stretching your legs out towards the front of the treadmill.
>
> The impact and the shock to your body will increase significantly with speed, and you will find that running fast becomes very hard work. This is the way most people run!

Remember: never try to increase your stride length by moving your foot forwards or by lifting your knee. This is also shown in illustrations 16 and 17 in Chapter 3, *Good technique—how it works*.

> EXERCISE 10.8: Accelerating by Increasing Your Cadence
>
> - Stand on the treadmill and start it at the lowest speed.
> - As the treadmill belt starts moving, start off at walking pace.
> - Gradually increase the speed of the treadmill and, as the belt speeds up, increase your cadence by stepping more quickly.
>
> Running along the ground like this will also prove to be very hard work and you will never reach your potential doing this.
>
> If your cadence is significantly higher at higher speeds than at lower speeds then you are not flying: you merely have a fast 'walking' action.

Now let's compare those two techniques with the efficiency of gaining an acceleration by increasing your time off the ground.

EXERCISE 10.9: Accelerating by Getting Airborne

- Before you start the treadmill, stand in the middle of the belt and mark the position of your feet with some tape on the side of the treadmill.

  This is your landing spot. Make sure you land here throughout this exercise.

- With the treadmill belt still stationary, bounce on both feet and then progress to bounce on alternate your feet, as you did in EXERCISE 6.2.

- Start the treadmill, allowing the belt to travel under you while you bounce. Make sure that your heel touches down firmly.

  The landings will be heavy and noisy, especially until the belt speeds up.

- As the belt speeds up, spend a little more time off the ground by increasing the power of your take-off.

  Your foot will naturally land back under your hips, allowing you to use the natural elasticity in your legs to spring, and reduce the effort of leaving the ground.

  Your body will remain erect, and your action will be smooth and easy.

- Focus on landing level with your marked landing spot.

  While you are touching the belt, your foot will be pushed back, and your body will therefore be naturally tilted forwards. This means that all you need to do is focus on landing on the same spot each time and the rest will happen naturally.

When at constant speed:

- Once you have accelerated to a comfortable speed, keep landing on the same spot.

  This will give you a smooth and efficient running action at a constant speed.

- Continue running like this for some time.

    By continuing running like this for some time, you will be more likely to carry over this good running technique into all your runs.

    When you are ready to stop:

- As the belt slows down, continue to focus on your landing spot and reduce the power of your take-off.

    This will give you a controlled deceleration.

10.3 Summary

This chapter is all about carrying on the good work you have done in changing your technique. Your running has probably improved dramatically by now, but technique change is a long-term ongoing process.

You need to constantly check your running technique. It is easy to get complacent at this point, but you need to continue to apply a critical eye to all aspects of your running action.

You will need to pay attention to what you are doing in your training runs, and correct any faults as you become aware of them. The exercises in the first part (Section 10.1) of this chapter will give you some very good ways to do this.

Once you are comfortable with your running action, use the exercises and checks in the second part (Section 10.2) of this chapter to further refine your technique and make fine adjustments to it.

CHAPTER 11
HEIDI'S STRENGTHENING PROGRAM

Heidi Jones

Move over Keith, this is my turn! While Keith is concentrating on fixing your running action, my job is to help you strengthen your feet and glutes. Please don't neglect the exercises in this chapter, as strength in these two areas is vital if you want to run well.

Heidi's Strengthening Program consists of a series of exercises that I have developed to help you build up strength in both your feet and glutes. Most of the exercises in the program are devoted to the feet, as weakness here will result in weakness further up the body. The program gives you an effective way to handle technique change and to transition to lighter shoes; if you don't do it, you will almost certainly get injured. On the other hand, if you do happen to incur any injuries, either during your transition or afterwards, please refer to Chapter 13, *Heidi's rehabilitation exercises*.

Heidi's Strengthening Program consists of three stages:
- rolling out the plantar fascia
- exercising the foot
- exercising the glutes.

You start by rolling your feet over a hard spiky ball to loosen them up. Then, you do the Foot Program, which consists of five foot exercises and an ankle stretch, before finishing off with my Quarter Knee Squat to strengthen your glutes.

All stages of the program should be done daily.

The first two stages (the Spiky Ball and the Foot Program) focus on exercising the feet, as this is where you will experience the greatest change in use.

The third stage, the Quarter Knee Squat exercise, is specifically designed to develop your gluteus medius muscles, which you need for stability and upper-body support. Please note that my Quarter Knee Squat is different to the many similarly named variations shown on the Internet.

Each exercise in Heidi's Strengthening Program builds on the previous one, so make sure you move through the exercises sequentially. All the exercises in this chapter are suitable for runners and non-runners. You can see the videos of all my exercises on the olderyetfaster.com website.

For more details about the exercises from a medical perspective, see Appendix B, *For podiatrists—treating runners* and Appendix C, *Heidi's Strengthening Program explained*.

11.1 Strengthening your feet

As you transition to good form via Keith's Lessons, you will inevitably experience calf pain due to increased muscular use. I specially developed the Spiky Ball and Foot Program exercises to strengthen your feet and help deal with this calf pain.

These exercises also form a suitable rehabilitation program for Achilles tendonitis and tendinosis, and help relieve plantar fasciitis.

The Spiky Ball

For this exercise, you need a hard spiky ball of 10 centimetres in diameter to roll out the plantar fascia. I used to provide medium-density spiky balls for my clients, but I found that after a couple of weeks they became too soft and thus of little use. I recommend you purchase a hard, high-density ball like the ball pictured in *Illustration 36*, which is the same type that I use in my practice. It is available at sports stores and physio suppliers.

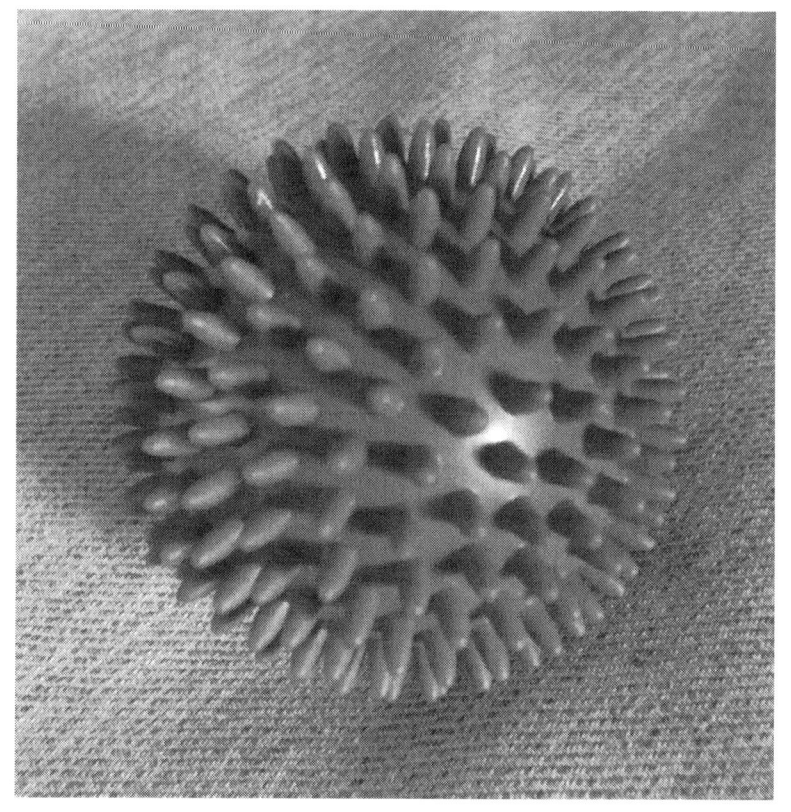

Illustration 36: *A hard high-density spiky ball—available at sports stores and physio suppliers. Make sure it is hard, spiky and about 10 centimetres in diameter. Photo by Stuart Greaves.*

At first, some people find using the spiky ball a bit harsh, but after a week or so they become accustomed to it and most come to love it. If you are like me and Keith, it will become your friend. Every time I use my spiky ball and do the Foot Program, my feet feel fantastic, like they have had a strong massage, and have had a thorough workout.

The Spiky Ball exercise is more effective if you do it standing up, because then it will also strengthen your gluteus medius muscle (glutes) on your weight-bearing leg.

Surprisingly, I have found that a large number of people struggle to stand on one leg due to their weak glutes. This weakness can most probably be attributed to constantly wearing shoes with a raised heel. For a demonstration of how to do the exercise, see my video via olderyetfaster.com.

You should be able to do this massage exercise for 3–5 minutes without fatiguing on the weight-bearing leg. It also gives a good indication of how strong or weak your feet and glutes are.

> EXERCISE 11.1: The Spiky Ball
>
> In this exercise you will roll your feet over a hard spiky ball. This will help to 'iron out' your plantar fascia (the thick fibrous band on the bottom of the foot running from the heel to the five toes) and make it supple. This is the most important exercise you need to do for your feet and calf muscles to remain injury free.
>
> Do this exercise before and after your run. Before a run it will help loosen your feet. After a run it will help with recovery.
>
> Ensure both your feet are facing forwards, hip-width apart.
>
> - Stand on one leg and place the spiky ball just in front, and to the side of, the big toe of your weight-bearing foot.
> - Place the heel of your non-weight-bearing foot on the spiky ball.
> - Roll the ball *hard* and *slow* to your toes and back again.
>
>   Always roll the ball under your body and lean slightly onto the ball for a firmer massage.
>
> - Roll the ball along the arch of your foot, then on the outer edge of your foot, always going full length both ways.
> - Repeat rolling the ball forwards and back for three to five minutes.
> - Then, repeat the exercise standing on your other foot.
>
> When you do this exercise, make sure that the pressure is always comfortable and enjoyable.
>
> If you are injured and it hurts to stand, you can still do this exercise from a sitting position to benefit your feet and calves.
>
> Thanks to Angelo Castiglione, founder of 180 Degrees Wellness, Leichhardt, Australia, for this exercise.

The Foot Program

Now that your feet are relaxed and supple, start to exercise the muscles of your feet with the Foot Program, which consists of the following exercises:

- The Maestro
- Birdie on a Wire
- Foot Bridges
- Toe Wave
- Marble Mover
- Front of Shin and Ankle Stretch.

The first five exercises should be done in sequence, and the entire set should take about 5 minutes. Remember to roll out your feet with the spiky ball before you start.

Do each of the Foot Program exercises ten times and finish off with the Front of Shin and Ankle Stretch exercise.

Take note of the exercises that you find challenging and focus on them. These will be the ones you need the most. The good news is that if you have found a weakness, you can work on it and fix it. If you feel sore after doing the exercises, this is an indication that you are extremely weak. If you do these exercises each day, within a couple of months your feet will be flexible and strong.

> EXERCISE 11.2: The Maestro—Conduct the Orchestra!
>
> The Maestro is an excellent exercise for strengthening your pronator and supinator muscles and tendons. It helps to rehabilitate nearly every foot ailment.
>
> The exercise will also provide relief from Morton's neuroma (a painful condition producing nerve pain in the ball of the foot, most commonly between the third and fourth toes) and relieve general foot pain, especially if you have worn tight or high-heeled shoes. It is also beneficial for straightening the big toe; this helps to fix early-stage bunions and thus makes the big toe less susceptible to arthritis.
>
> See *Illustration 37*.

- Sit on a chair and extend your legs, keeping your feet shoulder-width apart. See *Illustration 37*, position 1.

  Keep your knees pointing up towards the ceiling for the entire exercise. Do not rotate your legs. You should only be moving your feet and your ankles.

- Point your feet, then arc them in so your soles face each other (inversion). See *Illustration 37*, position 2.
- Hold and separate your toes for three seconds.
- Arc your feet out, going though position 1, so your soles face away from each other (eversion). Hold and separate your toes for three seconds. See *Illustration 37*, position 3.
- Repeat this exercise ten times.

Thanks to Pilates teacher Gaetano Del Monaco, Bondi Junction, Australia for this exercise.

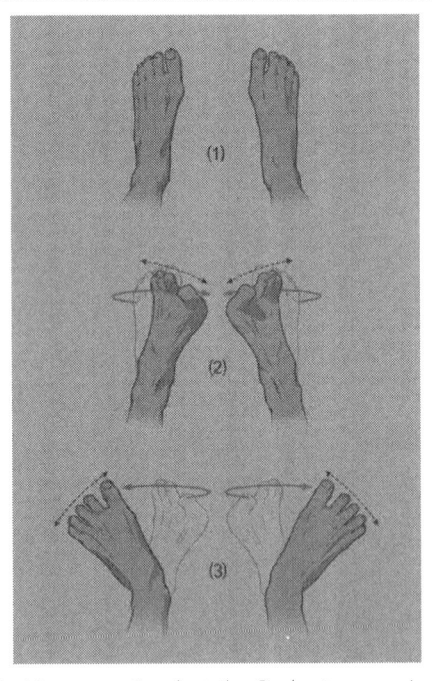

Illustration 37: *The Maestro—Conduct the Orchestra exercise. Positions 1 to 3.*

EXERCISE 11.3: Birdie on a Wire

If you cannot see your toe knuckles, they should reappear after working at this exercise, sometimes in one session. This exercise is great for misaligned toe knuckles (dropped metatarsal heads) and helps to prevent clawing of the toes, as well as prevent calluses and corns associated with clawed-toe deformity.

- Sit in a chair with both legs extended. See *Illustration 38*, position 1.

- Curl your toes. See *Illustration 38*, position 2.

  Can you see your toe knuckles (metatarsal heads)?

  Hold for two seconds.

- Point your feet, keeping your toes curled. See *Illustration 38*, position 3.

  Hold for two seconds.

- Dorsiflex your feet (move your feet towards your shins), keeping your toes curled. See *Illustration 38*, position 4.

  Hold for two seconds.

- Uncurl your toes and point them towards your body, fully stretching the underside of your toes, the soles of your feet and your calf muscles. See *Illustration 38*, position 5.

  Hold for five seconds.

- Repeat this exercise ten times.

If you can see your five toe knuckles, your toes are aligned. If you cannot see them, you will often see them appearing after you have done this exercise for a few weeks.

If you have extremely high-arched rigid feet, this might not happen, but the exercise is still very helpful in promoting strength and flexibility.

Thanks to Pilates teacher Gaetano Del Monaco, Bondi Junction, Australia for this exercise.

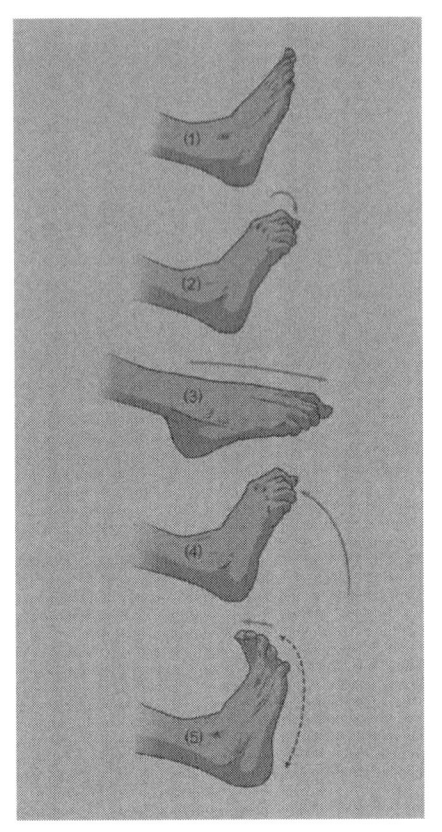

Illustration 38: Birdie on a Wire exercise. Positions 1 to 5.

EXERCISE 11.4: Foot Bridges

In the Foot Bridges exercise, you will continue to realign your toes with your toe knuckles and strengthen the three arches of your foot: medial longitudinal (inside), lateral longitudinal (outside), and transverse (across your forefoot).

You may find this exercise tricky: it involves a tiny movement that is isolated to the foot. It took me three weeks to be able to do it correctly. See *Illustration 39*.

- Sit on a chair. Keep your feet flat on the floor. See *Illustration 39*, position 1.

   Note the white stripe at the front of the shin in the illustration; this is your tibialis anterior tendon. Try to keep this relaxed as you do this exercise.

- Press the base of your toes into the floor. See *Illustration 39*, position 2.

  Only a tiny movement is required. Keep your toes straight. You should now be able to see your knuckles and feel a movement in the arch of your foot.

  If you gently place three fingers over your outer foot knuckles, you will feel them rise up as you press your toes into the floor.

- Repeat the exercise ten times.

If you find this exercise too difficult, practice picking up pegs or pens from the ground with your toes.

Thanks to Pilates teacher Gaetano Del Monaco, Bondi Junction, Australia for this exercise.

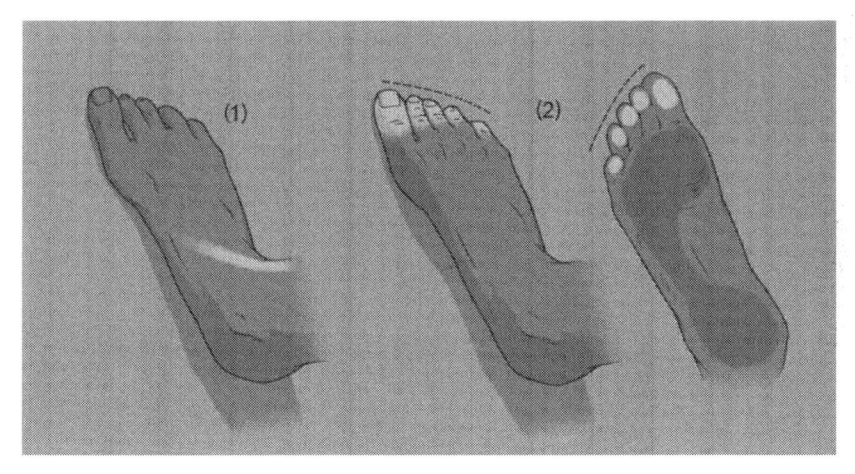

Illustration 39: Foot Bridges exercise. Positions 1 and 2.

EXERCISE 11.5: Toe Wave

This standing exercise follows on from the Foot Bridges exercise and is great for 'dropped toe knuckles'. Most importantly, it strengthens the intrinsic muscles of your forefoot, which play a major role in balance and maintaining the arch across your forefoot. It also stretches your plantar fascia and Achilles tendon, and works the tibialis anterior muscle (the stabilising muscle at the front of the shin that attaches to the foot) and tendon.

As with the Birdie on a Wire exercise, the Toe Wave exercise helps prevent clawed toes and gives you strength, flexibility and control in the forefoot. See *Illustration 40*.

- Stand with your weight on your back leg and with your knee slightly bent.

  This switches on your gluteus medius and makes this a glute stability exercise as well.

- Rest the heel of your forwards leg on the ground. See *Illustration 40*, position 1.
- Lift the top of your foot towards the shin (dorsiflex).
- Curl your toes down and hold for 2 seconds. See *Illustration 40*, position 2.
- Curl your toes up and separate them. Hold for 2 seconds. See *Illustration 40*, position 3.

  Stretch and extend your toes, hard and slow.

Do this exercise slowly and in a controlled manner.

- Repeat the whole exercise ten times while your foot remains flexed.

  You should be able to see your toe knuckles (unless you have a rigid, high-arched foot).

- Swap legs and repeat the exercise with the other foot.

Thanks to running coach Alan McCloskey, Newcastle, Australia for this exercise.

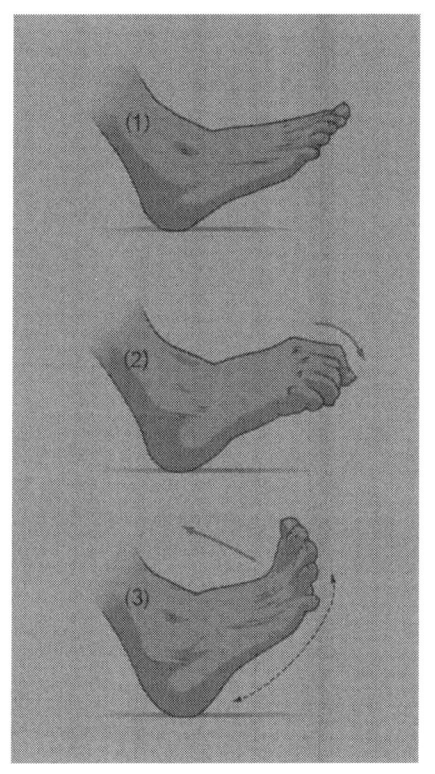

Illustration 40: Toe Wave exercise (standing toe curl). Positions 1 to 3.

EXERCISE 11.6: Marble Mover

In this standing exercise, you curl your toes as if picking up marbles, and then you turn your foot outward and uncurl your toes, stretching them upwards, as if dropping the marbles.

By doing this, you arch your foot, and this engages and strengthens both your tibialis posterior tendon and muscle. This is the key stabilising muscle of the lower leg and its tendon, which play a major role in supporting the medial arch of the foot.

This exercise also strengthens your arches, which you will need to get that rebound off the ground and run well. Once strong, you will never need supportive shoes or orthotics again. Freedom! See *Illustration 41*.

- Stand with your weight on your back leg.

  Your knee should be slightly flexed and your front leg should be resting with your heel on the ground. See *Illustration 41*, position 1.

- Pick up imaginary marbles with your toes.
- Lift your forefoot towards your shin (dorsiflex). See *Illustration 41*, position 2.
- Keeping your heel on the ground, turn your foot out half-way. See *Illustration 41*, position 3.

  Make sure you only turn your foot, not your hips.

- Drop the marbles. See *Illustration 41*, position 4.

  When you drop the marbles, fully stretch out, lifting your toes upwards and separating them.

- With your heel still on the ground, turn your foot back to position 1 and place your whole foot on the ground.

  This is the only time that your whole foot will be on the ground.

- Repeat this exercise ten times, and then change legs and repeat the exercise with the other foot.

Thanks to running coach Alan McCloskey, Newcastle, Australia for this exercise.

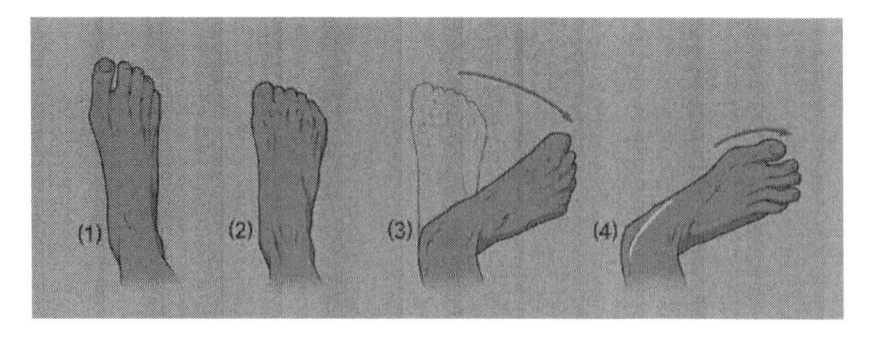

Illustration 41: Marble Mover exercise. Positions 1 to 4.

EXERCISE 11.7: Front of Shin and Ankle Stretch

This is a standing exercise.

The Front of Shin and Ankle Stretch opens up the front of the ankle joint and also releases the front of the shin muscle (the tibialis anterior). You will have worked this muscle hard in the previous exercises, so expect to feel tired in this area now.

People who complain of 'stiff ankles' really like these stretches as they increase ankle mobility. Surprisingly, the most common injury in this area is caused by shoe laces that are too tight!

This exercise will provide some relief as it releases the extensor tendons, which are on the top of the foot.

Do this stretch one foot at a time.

- Take a standing position.
- Place one leg slightly behind you with only the tips of your toes on the ground.
- Without moving your foot, pull your thigh forwards and feel an intense stretch at the front of your ankle. See *Illustration 42*, position 1.

  Hold for 15 seconds to open up the front of your ankle joint. This also stretches the front of your shin and your extensor tendons on the top of your foot.

- Intensify the stretch by rotating your foot out 90 degrees to the side, or as far as you can comfortably go. See *Illustration 43*, position 2.

  Hold for 15 seconds.

- Repeat this exercise with the other leg.

NOTE: If this stretch hurts your toes or you cannot feel it due to a toe deformity, roll up a towel and place it under your foot and try again.

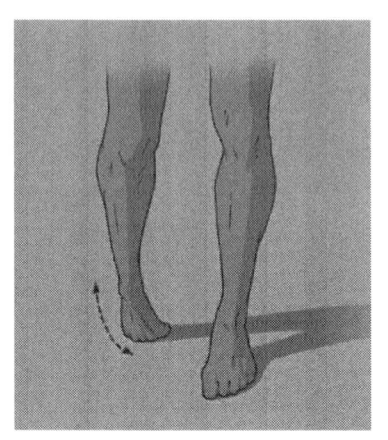

Illustration 42: Front of Shin and Ankle Stretch exercise. Position 1. stretch out the front of your shin, the top of your ankle and your extensor tendons.

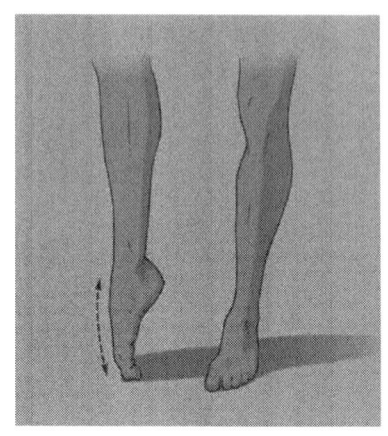

Illustration 43: Front of Shin and Ankle Stretch exercise. Position 2. to intensify the stretch, rotate your foot out 90 degrees.

This exercise completes my Foot Program. You just need to do my Quarter Knee Squat to complete Heidi's Strengthening Program.

11.2 Strengthening your glutes

If your glutes are weak (usually because of wearing shoes with a drop), you will be unstable and prone to injury. Your upper body needs firm support and the glutes keep your hips level and prevent your knees from collapsing inwards, which results in excessive pronation. Your glutes are also your powerhouse, which enables you to get your hips off the ground with minimum effort.

Even though your glutes will automatically strengthen as you stand and land aligned (OYF Rule #2), that will take time. My Quarter Knee Squat exercise will help with this.

Quarter Knee Squat

The Quarter Knee Squat exercise is especially important if you have weak glutes and are about to transition to running with good form.

EXERCISE 11.8: Quarter Knee Squat

The Quarter Knee Squat is a running-specific and weight-bearing exercise. It mimics that part of your running action where your foot is in full contact with the ground, but here there is no forwards component to your motion.

The reason this exercise is so beneficial is that, during the exercise, the gluteus medius, iliopsoas (hip flexor) and vastus medius obliquus (knee-stabilising muscle) work in unison, as they should when running.

- Stand upright in front of a full-length mirror.
- Place your hands on your hips.
- Slowly stand on one leg, keeping your knee in line with your second toe. See *Illustration 44*, position 1.

  If you are wobbling, then just do this until you become solid as a rock before moving on.

- Once you are not wobbling, slowly bend down so that your knee goes over your second toe, keeping your hips level and body upright (see *Illustration 44*, position 2). Do not bend forwards.

  Note that you are only going down approximately 8 centimetres (one quarter of the length of your shin bone) and no further.

- Slowly come back up to position 1.
- Start off with three sets of 10, and build up to three sets of 30 squats on each leg.

Once you get good at this exercise, incorporate it into your everyday life; for example, stand on one leg while chopping vegetables or cleaning your teeth. Make it fun!

And remember, as well as doing this exercise, you need to move to thin, flat and flexible shoes, since a raised heel in a shoe switches off your glutes, wasting all the effort you have put into making them strong.

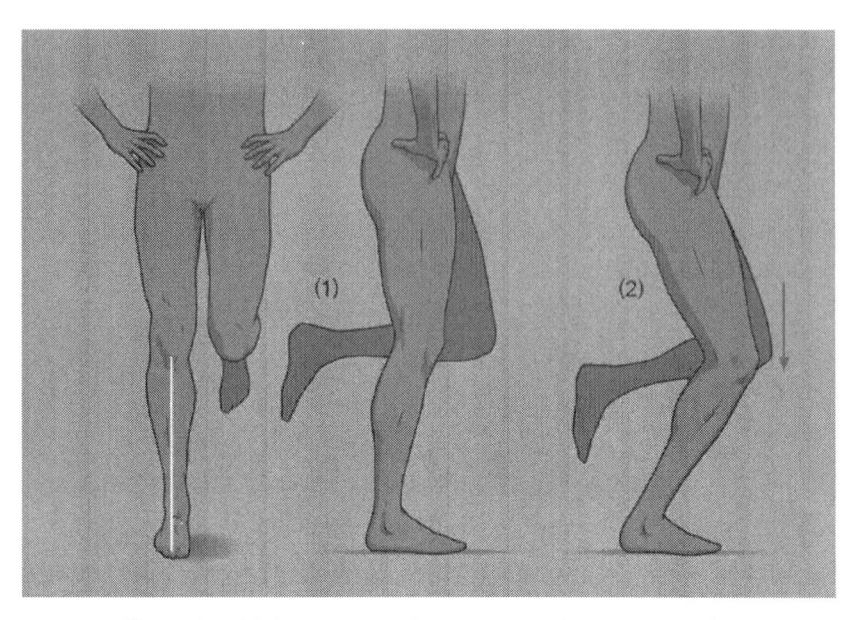

Illustration 44: Quarter Knee Squat exercise. Positions 1 and 2.

CHAPTER 12
MANAGING YOUR TRANSITION

Keith Bateman and Heidi Jones

If you follow Keith's Lessons in this book, you will transition to running with good technique. However, the transition will not happen overnight and you will experience many physical changes during this period, which usually lasts between 6 and 12 months. While you are transitioning, you will need to cut back on your training distances and refrain from any hard training. You will also need to adhere to *Heidi's Strengthening Program* (Chapter 11) to help you build up and reduce the chance of injury.

In this chapter, we look a bit closer at the changes you can expect during this transition period and identify stages you will go through.

12.1 Changes to expect

You might find the physical changes during transition unsettling at first—but think about the rewards. Your improved technique will allow you to run faster with less effort, and with a reduced weekly mileage. Then you can rebuild training distances and intensity to reach your full potential. You will also burn more fat, leading to a great body shape: if you want a six-pack and a tight butt, this is the way to get them!

Once your technique change has started to take effect, you will start to feel good about your running and you will experience regular speed improvements. You will probably also notice that you get out of breath more quickly. This is not a problem as you are just building new muscle and oxygen is being redirected to these areas.

Also expect to feel some soreness in your feet and legs—this will pass as you complete your transition to good form. Your lower legs will feel sore due to changing your running action and your footwear, while your feet will feel sore as you have started some barefoot running. Any calf muscle soreness may continue for a while and some clients report that it can be over six months before this soreness goes away.

The good news is that not only will you feel healthier and stronger, but your whole posture will improve and you will move and walk more easily. Your postural muscles will engage more fully and your core will strengthen. You will feel your muscles toning up and this definition will become apparent to your friends and family. You are likely to get compliments such as 'Have you been working out?', and 'Your calf muscles are looking cut'. As we have pointed out before in the book, you don't need to go to the gym to build up your body and your core strength. What you do need to pay attention to are the other changes in your body. As soon as you notice any weakness or pain, stop and make sure to go back to Heidi's Strengthening Program and build up these areas.

12.2 The stages of the transition

As you implement the OYF Running technique to learn to run correctly, you will find that you will move through stages during transition. We have identified three separate stages: Early Days, Muscle Rebuilding, and Reaping the Benefits.

In the Early Days stage, you will experience muscle soreness and will not be able to run long distances. You will know that you have moved on to the Muscle Rebuilding stage when you have stopped noticing muscle soreness and you are able to run longer distances. When you can regularly find your perfect balance point and get that magic rebound, you will have reached the final, Reaping the Benefits stage, and your running will suddenly take off to a new level.

These stages are discussed in more detail below.

Early Days stage

In the Early Days stage, your changed technique will not feel natural or even comfortable, but it will gradually become normal. Remember that your body will be making some major adjustments as you develop different muscle groups.

If you are a member of a running group, or you run with friends, we suggest that you run on your own for a while so that you can train at your own pace during this stage. At the beginning, aim for three runs per week, and start with no more than two kilometres; if you are new to running, do not worry if it is only 800 metres in your first few runs.

We recommend running on firm grass during this phase; the uneven ground will strengthen your feet. Short, but ever-increasing barefoot sessions, are the best way to learn. Running tracks are also good places to practice in the Early Days stage.

Muscle Rebuilding stage

You will know that you have moved on to the Muscle Rebuilding stage when you have stopped noticing muscle soreness and you are able to run longer distances. The Muscle Rebuilding stage is your strengthening and muscle rebuilding time, where you can start to introduce some speed sessions.

Although you will remain in this stage for some time, it does give you the opportunity to refine your technique.

Continue to monitor your form using the exercises in Chapter 10, *Lesson Six: Maintaining good form*, and make the necessary adjustments. You will find that, just by running well, you have been building muscle throughout your body in readiness for the final stage of your transition.

During the Muscle Rebuilding stage, you are likely to suffer a few setbacks, such as sore arches in your feet, or strained Achilles tendons or calf muscles. This is quite common, as it is very difficult to manage a perfectly-controlled body rebuild. Expect some delays, but remember these are just because your body is adapting. A little time spent on rehabilitation should leave the affected area in great shape for the future. If you are thinking of running a marathon, then allow for at least two years of strengthening.

Heidi says that tendon strength comes after muscular strength, so the Muscle Rebuilding stage is the period where your Achilles tendons and posterior tibial tendons will also be strengthening. If you get soreness in these areas, do not be discouraged. Stop running, do the exercises in

Heidi's Strengthening Program and resume training when you are pain free. Tendons respond to gentle loading and will recover.

Your progress will be much more rapid once you have good strength in your feet and legs. Speed will come first, then endurance. You will also find that you will be naturally running at 5 minutes per kilometre, or faster, at the end of a 3-kilometre warm-up. This is an excellent indication that everything is going to plan. Around this time of your training, people will have started to notice your stomach and your glutes tightening up.

When you can comfortably run 5 kilometres on the road, it is probably time to re-join your running group and start doing some speed work. Once you are used to racing and can run 5 kilometres in well under 25 minutes, you can think about some longer races of up to 10 kilometres. But don't get carried away: no half-marathons or marathons just yet. When you do run longer races, make sure that you always try to run with good form, and that you gradually increase your race distance. And do not make the mistake of thinking your transition is over just because you are racing. There is so much more to come!

Reaping the Benefits stage

During the Reaping the Benefits stage, the magic happens. You will find that you are suddenly running faster. This is because you have extended your stride length by getting slightly higher off the ground.

You will not notice the change until you check your watch. The reason you do not notice is that you are hardly braking at all and your precise near-vertically-aligned landings allow the elasticity in your legs to give you that extra lift (OYF Rule #4).

It is truly astonishing what improvement this minute change in balance has. 'It felt effortless, like I was flying' is a typical comment from clients when they reach this stage.

12.3 Main points to look out for in your transition

The following list summarises the main points to keep in mind during your training and all three stages of your transition.

- **Do the exercises in Heidi's Strengthening Program (Chapter 11)**
  In order to lessen the chance of incurring overuse injuries, you need to build up the necessary strength in your feet, calves and glutes. The best approach is to spend six weeks doing Heidi's strengthening exercises before you embark on your transition. Do the Spiky Ball and Foot Program exercises and Quarter Knee Squats daily. Continue with Heidi's Strengthening Program on your non-running days during your transition until you have no soreness.

- **Gradually build up training distance and intensity**
  If you are a seasoned runner, cut down your normal training program when you start the transition to OYF Running. Leave at least a day between runs, more if you have sore muscles. Treat your transition as if you are starting a new sport. If you have a history of foot or lower-leg injuries, proceed with extra caution. If you do suffer an injury during the transition, do not try to battle on. Refer to Heidi's Strengthening Program (Chapter 11) or refer to Chapter 13, *Heidi's rehabilitation exercises* and get the problem fixed before continuing. Once your feet and calf muscles have adapted, you can gradually build up to longer distances.

- **Review side-view videos**
  Be sure to continue to get side-view videos of your running action. This will help you determine what you are actually doing; many people think they've got it right, when in fact further work is needed (OYF Rule #1).

- **Determine the cause of any injuries**
  If you become injured, stop running and refer to chapter 13, Heidi's rehabilitation exercises. While you are resting, it is important to work out what caused it. Start your search by referring to Chapter 2, *Poor technique causes injuries,* and see if you can identify your symptoms in the list. If you have taken a side-on video of yourself before your injury, study your running action and see if you can identify the corresponding fault in your technique (OYF Rule #1). Chapter 13, *Heidi's rehabilitation exercises* covers the transitional soreness that you will encounter.

- **Get the right shoes**

    Shoe construction influences everything: your stance, your balance, your muscle use, your stress points, your technique, and eventually your body shape. This topic is very important and covered in much more detail in Chapter 14, *Shoes—what you need to know*.

> Personal story—Transition works
>
> David Blackman is a runner with Southampton Athletic Club (UK). After reading the first edition of *Older Yet Faster* he, with the help of his coach John Tilt, changed his technique. This is his experience in his own words:
>
>> 'Patience is absolutely essential, and the more carefully you progress, the fewer potential problems you will be exposed to, and the greater the rewards will be. For best results, I recommend that you suspend your racing program or chasing those personal records for a few months, and start running slowly to get that gait nailed. Exactly how many months this takes depends on how drastic a change you are making. For me, I had 37 years of very bad over-striding to undo, so I found that the back-to-basics, slower-paced phase [Early Days stage] took about nine months, followed by another four months of easing on the speed [Muscle Rebuilding stage].
>>
>> For long periods I was questioning the potential for success! But, for those runners requiring less dramatic changes, you may find you have successfully changed your basic style in two or three months, and added new speed by the time you reach four or five months. In one sentence: Start slow, be patient; later, ease on the speed gently'.
>
> For David, big improvements started to happen after 15 months [Reaping the Benefits stage]:
>
>> 'Four days after my fiftieth birthday, and 15 months after starting the Bateman–Jones journey [OYF Running], I equalled my 5 kilometre personal best/personal record from almost ten years earlier (16:37). In the same month, I also ran within 20 seconds of my 10 mile personal best/personal record (58:04), which I set in 1990 at the age of 23.'
>
> Three years after starting his transition, David is still improving. At the age of 51, on 11 March 2018, he ran a lifetime best 800 metres in 2:07.64.

CHAPTER 13
HEIDI'S REHABILITATION EXERCISES

Heidi Jones

In the course of your transition, you will naturally experience muscle soreness, which will mostly be in your calves and feet. This soreness can be easily managed by adjusting your training program, resting and doing some suitable exercises. There should be no need to consult a medical professional at this stage, but if you do, please ensure that they understand the physics of good running and will not be hindering your progress by advising supportive or cushioned shoes, or issuing orthotics.

However, if you do too much too soon, you might experience more serious injuries, such as calf tears or Achilles tendon problems. Tendons are the last structure to strengthen. Due to having received continued support, typically, people transitioning out of orthotics will be weaker in the tibialis posterior tendon (the tendon of the key stabilising muscle of the lower leg that attaches to the medial arch of the foot and is located at the back and to the inside of the shin bone), and therefore more prone to injury. If you need to warm up any sore tendon, do not be fooled into running, as this will still be causing damage and will extend your recovery time.

In this chapter, I not only discuss the differences between transitional soreness and more serious injuries, but I also suggest exercises for general rehabilitation.

13.1 Transitional soreness

Illustration 45 shows areas of the foot and lower leg that will come more into play due to your technique and shoe changes.

Sore calf muscles (*Illustration 45.1*) and foot arches (*Illustration 45.2*) are to be expected, and soreness means you are using your calves and feet more, and that they are strengthening. It can take 6 to 12 months for calf muscles to become comfortable with the new work load. You may need two or three days off between runs at the beginning. You need to be extremely patient, otherwise you can tear these muscles.

Achilles tendon soreness (*Illustration 45.3*) is not unusual and will happen if you do too much too soon. Press on the Achilles tendon with your fingers. This area should not be sore to touch and, if it is, you should not run; although you can usually keep the blood flowing with swimming, cycling or 10 minutes of easy walking.

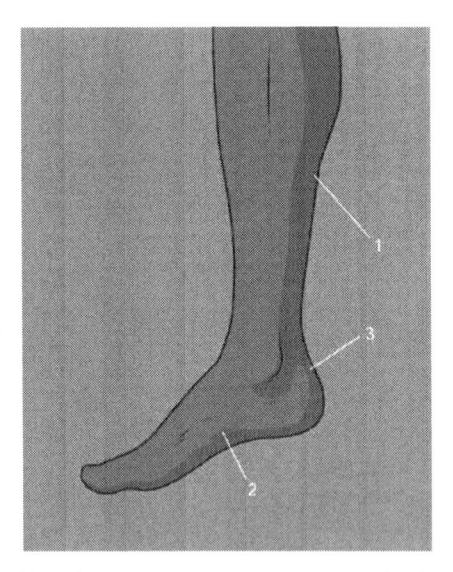

Illustration 45: Transitional soreness you may get as your body gets used to different pressures. This soreness will most commonly occur in the calves (1), foot arches (2) and Achilles tendons (3).

The endurance Straight Leg – Bent Leg Calf Raise exercise, which I describe in the next section, will help in the strengthening process.

Rolling your feet out with The Spiky Ball (see EXERCISE 11.1) will relieve the soreness in your feet, Achilles tendon and your calf muscles.

If you have persistent calf pain, check that you are not over-working your calf muscles by pushing hard off your forefoot. If you are doing this, there will probably be a callus build-up under your forefoot due to shearing forces. Try dorsiflexing your back foot as it leaves the ground, as mentioned in the *Beach check* and the *Dusty-track check* in Section 10.2.

If an injury keeps you awake at night, is stiff in the morning, or you notice it when not running, then you have a problem and you should stop running.

13.2 More serious injuries

This section deals with common injuries, such as more substantial calf and Achilles tendon soreness and tears, plantar fasciitis, runner's knee, and ankle and forefoot pain. These are generally caused by poor running technique and poor footwear choices rather than transitioning to an improved technique. However, as mentioned above, calf and Achilles tendon problems can also be caused by transitioning too quickly.

If you experience a more serious injury, the first thing to do is to stop running, rest from all painful activities and follow Heidi's rehabilitation exercises. While you are on the sidelines, it is also important to find the cause, so you can fix the problem and not just the symptom (OYF Rule #6). Start by studying Chapter 2, *Poor technique causes injuries*, to work out why you have the injury. When you are fully healed, remember to check your form by taking videos frequently (OYF Rule #1): make sure your heel firmly touches the ground during constant-speed running. Also check your shoes, which are frequently the cause of an injury (see Chapter 14).

Achilles tendon injuries

A sore Achilles tendon is commonly caused by wearing a soft, spongy shoe: the shoe makes you unstable and stresses the tendon as it sinks and twists on each landing. This injury is also caused by toe-running—check if you have calluses on your forefoot or toes. If soreness is caused by transitioning, it is usually due to insufficient recovery between runs—getting excited and doing too much, too soon.

I rehabilitate a sore Achilles tendon by using the Straight Leg – Bent Leg Calf Raise exercise (see *Illustration 46*) after doing the Spiky Ball and Foot Program. The Straight Leg – Bent Leg Calf Raise exercise builds endurance and strength in your calf muscles and Achilles tendons.

Start strengthening both tendons with EXERCISE 13.1 (see below), as tendons respond well to gentle loading. We are strengthening both Achilles tendons initially, as we don't want to overload them.

If you are not wearing thin, flat, flexible shoes, then do so now, as there is nothing more stable than the ground. Wearing soft spongy footwear will only aggravate the tendon, as it sinks and twists with every step. If you are unable to manage your pain with rest or with the exercises in this book, you will need to seek advice from your medical professional. However, as mentioned above, do keep it simple and do not change your biomechanics with unsuitable shoes or orthotics.

EXERCISE 13.1: Straight Leg – Bent Leg Calf Raise

The Straight Leg – Bent Leg Calf Raise exercise is only needed if you are coming back from a calf tear or an Achilles tendon injury.

If you have a calf tear, you need to rest from all painful activity. Start rehabilitation once you can walk pain free.

If you have Achilles tendonitis, you can begin rehabilitation immediately, as tendons respond to gentle loading. Start off conservatively and reassess the following day.

Refer to *Illustration 46* for this exercise.

- On flat ground, lightly hold a bench or wall for balance.
- Rise up onto the balls of your feet (*Illustration 46*, left figure) and hold this position for 45 seconds.
- Slowly bend your knees (*Illustration 46*, right figure) and hold for another 45 seconds. (That is one set.)

  Start with one set daily and work up to doing three consecutive sets of this exercise, for a total of four and a half minutes.

- When you can do this exercise daily for one week, progress to doing this exercise on one leg.

> Remember to start off with one set and build up to three consecutive sets. This will give you strength and endurance in your calf muscles, and strengthen your Achilles tendons.
>
> When you can do this exercise all the way through on one leg without pain recurring the next day and you can press firmly on your Achilles tendon with no pain, stop the calf raise. You are now ready to strengthen your glutes by resuming my Quarter Knee Squat (EXERCISE 11.8).
>
> Start off with three sets of 10 and work up to three sets of 30 on each leg. This is because glute weakness can cause excessive hip-drop leading to over-pronation, which in turn stresses the Achilles tendon. Once you can do this, you are ready to resume running.
>
> Start back conservatively, i.e. run 2 kilometres every second day for the first week.
>
> Thanks to Dr Chris Jones, osteopath and runner, Bondi Junction, Australia for this exercise.

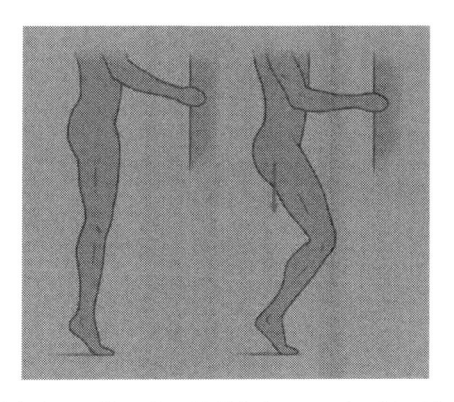

Illustration 46: Straight Leg – Bent Leg Calf Raise exercise (double-leg version shown). Rise up onto the balls of your feet (left) and hold this position for 45 seconds. Slowly bend your knees (right) and hold for another 45 seconds.

Calf tears

If you have torn your calf muscle, you need to stop and rest and may even need crutches if it hurts to walk. Wearing a compression sleeve will help support the muscle. Don't start rehabilitation until you are able to walk without pain. This can take weeks, so be patient. Twenty minutes of ice applied to the area, and resting with your leg elevated helps with recovery and pain relief.

When you can walk pain free, do my Spiky Ball and Foot Program exercises, and then do the Straight Leg – Bent Leg Calf Raise (EXERCISE 13.1) daily. Start off on both legs and stop as soon as your calf muscles start to fatigue (this may be less than one set). Slowly build up to three sets, with a break between each set. Then build up to three sets without a break.

When you can do three consecutive sets daily for one week, progress to the single leg version of this exercise. Since you cannot run, you might as well take this opportunity to strengthen both calf muscles, so do the exercises on each leg. Again, do three sets with a break in between, and slowly build up to three consecutive sets. When you can do this for one week, stop the calf exercise and resume my Quarter Knee Squat exercise (EXERCISE 11.8). Start off with three sets of 10, and work up to three sets of 30. Do this daily for one week. Now you are ready to run.

Plantar fasciitis

Plantar fasciitis is a common, painful disorder affecting the heel and the underside of the foot.

The following Plantar Fascia Stretch exercise is only needed if you are recovering from plantar fasciitis and is to be done after my Spiky Ball and the Foot Program exercises. It is not recommended if you have bunions or a toe deformity.

If your shoes have a raised heel and turned-up toe box, be sure to change them to thin, flat, flexible shoes to relieve the stress on the plantar fascia. See Chapter 2, *Poor technique causes injuries*.

Recovering from plantar fasciitis can take several months, depending on the severity. Do not run until it is completely healed. Also, don't do any other activity that produces pain after or the following day. Sufferers will also benefit from putting the injured foot into a bucket of hot water for 10 minutes before rolling out their foot, as this will help break up scar tissue. When you are pain free, resume the Quarter Knee Squat exercise (EXERCISE 11.8) daily. Start off with three sets of 10 and work up to three sets of 30. Do this daily for one week and then you are ready to run.

EXERCISE 13.2: Plantar Fascia Stretch

This is an intense stretch unless you already have very flexible feet.

Refer to *Illustration 47*.

- If required, hold on to a table or bench for balance.
- From a standing position, bend your knees so you are squatting, with your calf muscles touching your hamstrings.
- Slowly lower your knees to the ground and sit upright.
- Hold the position for as long as you can, up to 20 seconds.
- Always follow this stretch with the Front of Shin and Ankle Stretch (EXERCISE 11.7, see *Illustration 42* and *Illustration 43* in Chapter 11, *Heidi's Strengthening Program*).

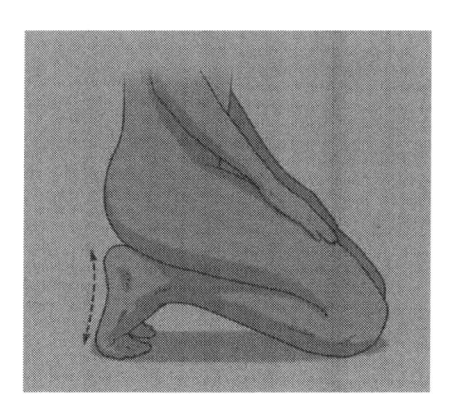

Illustration 47: *Plantar Fascia Stretch exercise.*

Knee problems

The knee joint is under a great deal of pressure in all directions when over-striding and when wearing shoes with a drop, and under medial pressure when wearing orthotics or 'supportive' shoes. Common knee injuries are runner's knee and medial meniscus pain.

Runner's knee (see also Section 2.2, *Injuries to the rest of the body*) is a technique-related injury and should disappear with improved technique. However, do not attempt to run until you are completely pain free. You must get into thin, flat, flexible shoes immediately to take the pressure off the knee joint.

Medial meniscus pain is pain located on the inner side of the knee joint and is almost always associated with wearing orthotics or supportive footwear. Treatment of medial meniscus pain is by pronating the foot, which usually just means removing any orthotic and getting the patient into thin, flat, flexible footwear.

For both conditions, it is important for sufferers to stabilise the knees by strengthening the vastus medialis obliquus (VMO) muscle using EXERCISE 13.3. The VMO is the pear-shaped muscle just above, and to the inside of, the knee. This is the main knee-stabilising muscle of the thigh muscles (quadriceps). You might have to work through a little bit of pain at first. This is the only exercise where this is the case.

For knee injury pain relief, and to facilitate healing by increasing blood flow, alternate 20 minutes heat applied to the injured area of the knee with 20 minutes of ice applied to the same area, followed by another 20 minutes of heat. Always start and finish with heat. You must stop running immediately. Do my Spiky Ball and Foot Program exercises daily and then do the Fixing Runner's Knee and Medial Meniscus Pain exercise (EXERCISE 13.3). Do three sets of 20 each morning and evening. Depending of the severity, your injury can take up to nine months to fully heal. When you are pain free, resume my Quarter Knee Squat (EXERCISE 11.8) daily. Start off with three sets of 10 and work up to three sets of 30. Do this daily for one week and then you are ready to run.

EXERCISE 13.3: Fixing Runner's Knee and Medial Meniscus Pain

You will need an adjustable ankle weight (or a towel over the top of your foot and a bucket with water in it). Start off with an ankle weight (see *Illustration 48*) of 2 kilograms (2 litres of water) and work up to 3 kilograms.

This exercise is designed to strengthen your VMO muscle. Strengthening this muscle will help you to regain muscle balance so your kneecap once again tracks correctly.

The most benefit will be gained by doing this exercise in a slow and controlled manner. Refer to *Illustration 49*.

- Sit on a bench.

  Ensure your spine is neutral: not too erect, not slouching. Make sure your legs are hanging off the ground.

- Put your thumb on the VMO of the leg that has the weight on it.

- Point your foot towards your shin (dorsiflexion, see *Illustration 49*, position 1) and slowly extend your leg, but do not fully straighten it (*Illustration 49*, position 2).

  Feel the VMO working.

- Hold your foot in the dorsiflexed position.

- Stop and then point your foot (*Illustration 49*, position 3).

- Flex your foot back again (foot to shin) (*Illustration 49*, position 4).

- Keeping your foot flexed, bring your leg slowly back down (*Illustration 49*, position 5).

- Repeat the above steps three times without straightening your leg.

- Then, after the third leg extension, straighten your leg all the way.

- Do a total of 20 leg extensions.

Do three sets of 20 leg extensions with the weight on each leg, twice daily.

If you are recovering from runner's knee, iliotibial band friction syndrome or any injury further up the body (for example, hip flexor pain), then my Quarter Knee Squat (EXERCISE 11.8) is advised once the knee is pain free.

Thanks to Pilates teacher Gaetano Del Monaco, Bondi Junction, Australia for this exercise.

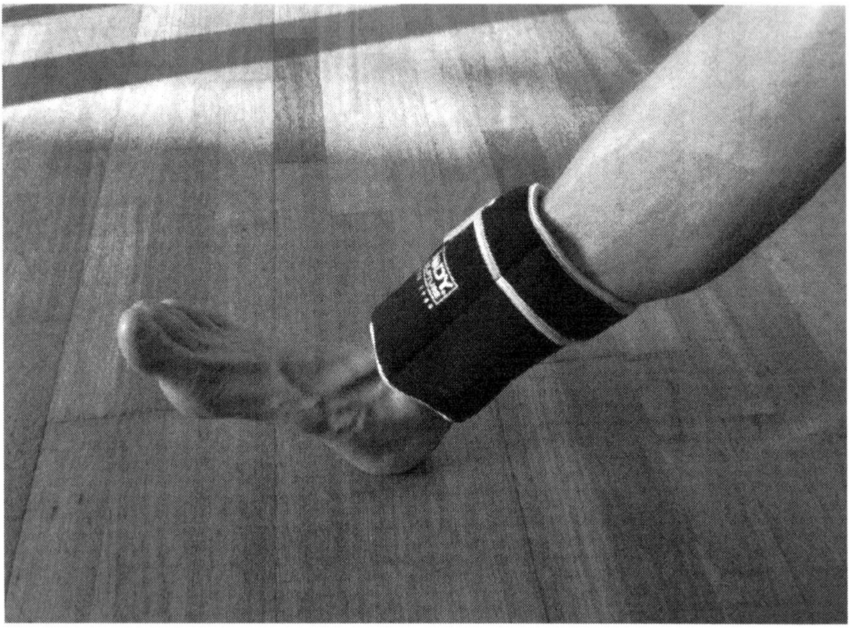

Illustration 48:. Adjustable ankle weight used in the Fixing Runner's Knee and Medial Meniscus Pain exercise. Photo by Stuart Greaves

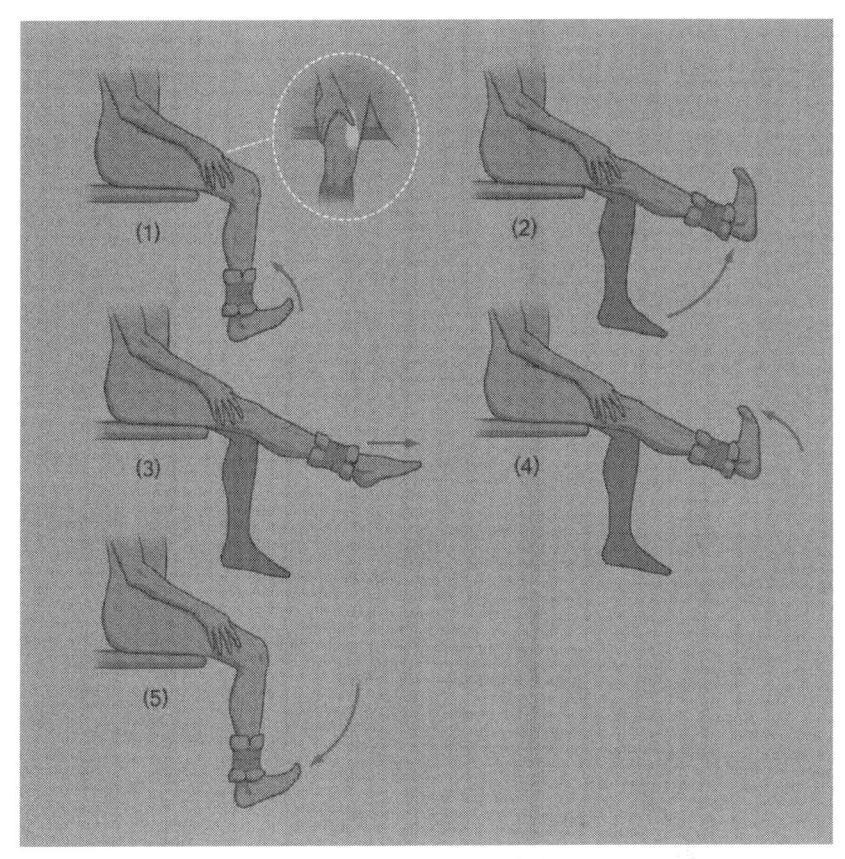

Illustration 49: Fixing Runner's Knee and Medial Meniscus Pain exercise. Positions 1 to 5.

Ankle pain

Pain under the ankle bone, either on the outside (peroneal tendonitis) or the inside of the foot (posterior tibial tendonitis), is usually due to excessive pronation as a result of over-striding. If you have not twisted your ankle and you do not also have calf pain, then over-striding is almost certainly the cause of your ankle pain.

To begin your recovery, you need to stop running and do my Spiky Ball and Foot Program exercises (see Section 11.1, *Strengthening your feet*). You might need to roll out your feet in a seated position until you are able to bear weight without pain and can progress to doing the exercise standing up. Then, when you can stand on one leg without pain, progress to doing my Quarter Knee Squat (EXERCISE 11.8) as well. Start off with three sets of 10 and work up to three sets of 30. When you can do this pain free daily for one week, you are ready to resume running.

Once you have recovered, you need to repeat Keith's Lessons to improve your technique and avoid this injury.

Forefoot pain

Forefoot pain is always due to poor technique. If you have calluses on your toes or on your forefoot, or if your shoes are wearing anywhere on the forefoot, then you are applying a dangerous amount of pressure to this area. Continuing with this bad form of running can lead to foot injuries, such as metatarsal stress fractures, Achilles tendonitis, peroneal tendonitis, and knee pain (see Chapter 2, *Poor technique causes injuries*).

If you have this pain, stop running and do my Spiky Ball and Foot Program exercises daily. If you can stand without pain, also do my Quarter Knee Squat (EXERCISE 11.8) daily. Start off with three sets of 10 and work up to three sets of 30. If you have pain when you stand, gently roll your foot over the spiky ball in a seated position, and wait until you can stand pain free before doing it in a standing position. Now you can also resume my Quarter Knee Squat exercise. Continue doing both exercises daily until your symptoms have resolved.

When you have recovered, you need to take a side-view video (OYF Rule #1) to recognise what you are doing. Then, go through the lessons again, paying particular attention to what your landings feel like. Barefoot running on a hard surface will be particularly useful and make you feel what is happening during each landing.

CHAPTER 14
SHOES—WHAT YOU NEED TO KNOW

Keith Bateman and Heidi Jones

If you have followed Keith's Lessons, then by now you should be feeling good about your running. However, it would be a shame to come this far and undermine all your hard-won progress by choosing the wrong shoes. We know you probably have your favourite shoes, but if they are unsuitable, then you are not going to reach your potential and you could injure yourself.

Nature provides you with a solid platform to stand, walk and run on. Each of your feet has 26 bones; over 100 muscles, tendons and ligaments; 33 joints and numerous blood vessels and nerves. These complex structures work efficiently together to interact with the ground to provide you with balance, support, propulsion and, in good runners, a large amount of spring. No shoe manufacture could possibly compete with this.

The obstruction or failure of any part in your feet can result in problems elsewhere in the body. Putting anything between your feet and the ground will alter your biomechanics and the way you run. Shoe construction influences everything: your stance, your balance, your muscle use, your stress points, your technique and, eventually, your body shape. Poorly designed shoes put your body out of alignment and are the biggest obstacle to good running technique and, in our opinion, the main contributor to running injuries and long-term skeletal damage.

To interfere as little as possible with your naturally efficient running, you need to use the flattest, thinnest and most flexible shoes that your current skill level will allow.

14.1 'Technology' in shoes is never beneficial

You probably thought that, although you had something to learn about how to run better, you still knew what was important in a running shoe. Surprisingly, most of you will be completely wrong thinking this. The compelling myth is that for running shoes to be any good they must have a host of modern technological features; that is, heavy cushioning, support, and should slope from heel to toe. This long-standing belief has become firmly entrenched, but we hope you will see through it by the end of this chapter, and that you will come to recognise what is really important in a running shoe.

Over decades, shoe companies have waged a dedicated and inexorable campaign to indoctrinate generations of walkers and runners with their unfounded advertising propaganda. Since the introduction of modern technology in shoe design in the late 1970s, race times for most groups of runners have been slower and injury rates have been higher. Also, previously rare injuries are now common. We attribute this, and most foot problems, almost exclusively to these 'modern' shoes.

What adults, and especially children, actually need is to walk and run in thin, flat, flexible shoes. These allow the natural foot action, which strengthens their young feet and bodies, rather than weaken them. In South Africa some schools recognise this and insist that children train barefoot for all school sports. In fact, the South African National Guidelines on School Uniforms lists footwear as 'optional'. Unfortunately, in Australia, some schools punish children for *not* wearing shoes that have 'support' and a heel!

In mainstream media, ideas such as cushioning and raised heels seem to have come from the misguided belief that they will provide comfort and pain relief for people who have been running badly. Unfortunately, these shoe 'enhancements' simply allow those people to run badly for longer, causing more stress, which might not become apparent until more serious injuries put a stop to running or lead to surgical intervention. Other assertions about shoes are propped up by questionable biomechanical theories that are now being superseded by theories that take into account the foot in action. Heidi covers this more fully in Appendix B, *For podiatrists—treating runners*.

14.2 Our guide to shoes

In our guide to shoes, we start off by describing what to look for in a shoe and what features to avoid, and we illustrate these in the diagrams. We then go on to explain the importance of these features and how badly designed shoes will affect your performance and can result in injuries. Poor shoes will affect your running action; and we give the reasons why you need the right shoes to maintain optimal performance. Finally, we go into detail about how the use of orthotics to fix defects in your running action will not help and why it will have adverse effects on your body.

What to look for in a shoe

All you need in a shoe is protection from dangerous objects, rough surfaces, temperature extremes, and a little extra cushioning for running on harder surfaces and when you are tired. Running on the road in a shoe should feel almost as good as running barefoot on a running track. If it does not, then there is a problem with your shoes, your technique or both. The shoe must also comfortably accommodate the shape of your foot. With today's modern materials this means, at most, 10 millimetres of sole and a comfortable upper that holds the shoe firmly to your foot. See *Illustration 50*.

The right shoe is vital for good running technique, but unfortunately there are not many of these shoes on the market, as there is little profit to be made out of selling such a simple product. We have checked shops across the UK, the US and Australia, and the worst place to buy shoes for running appears to be the running section of mainstream stores. Nevertheless, good shoes can be found, so do persevere. Sometimes you will have better luck with gym or cross-fit shoes.

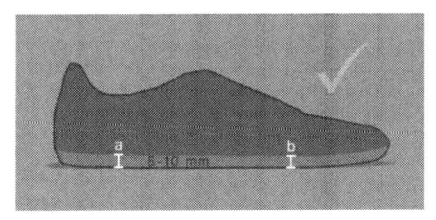

Illustration 50: *Features of a good shoe. The right shoe has a 5-10 mm thin (a) and (b) sole, which is flat and flexible and provides a little cushioning and protection from heat, cold and rough ground.*

Features of a good shoe

A good shoe (*Illustration 50*) should:

- be thin: a 5-10 millimetres sole should be ample in all conditions (*Illustration 50*, *a* and *b*)—you should be able to feel the ground
- be flat: there should be no raised heel (no 'drop' from heel to toe; see *Illustration 50*, *a* equals *b*)
- be flexible: the shoe should mimic the pliability of the feet, so you should be able to uniformly bend and twist the shoe in your hands—it should curl evenly and it should not have a hard plastic sole as some 'minimalist' shoes have
- have a wide toe box: your toes should have room to move
- have no arch support: pronation is a vital part of your suspension
- have the same sole material all over: no different density materials and no splits or cavities—they are stone-catchers!
- be light: why lift more than you need to?

These principles also apply to everyday shoes. Wearing good everyday shoes will straighten your whole body for running and will probably relieve any knee, hip, back or neck pain from poor footwear. If you start getting sore calf muscles, that is good! It simply means your calf muscles are strengthening; so just make sure you continue with caution while they build up.

The American College of Sports Medicine also provides good information on shoe choice. It is consistent with our own ideas. See their website at www.acsm.org.

Features of a bad shoe

The wrong shoe applies extra pressures to your foot and stops it working the way it should, which in turn stresses the rest of the body.

A bad shoe (*Illustration 51*) has at least one of these features:

- an unnecessarily thick and soft sole at the rear of the shoe (*Illustration 51.a*)
- an unnecessarily thick sole under the midfoot (*Illustration 51.b*)
- a drop: the shoe slopes from heel to toe (*Illustration 51.c*)

- a flared heel (*Illustration 51.d*): the back of the sole slopes outward
- a stiff or angled heel counter (*Illustration 51.e*)
- a turned-up toe box area (*Illustration 51.f*).
- a stiff sole: either the whole sole or part of it
- an arch support—a 'stability' shoe
- a narrow toe box
- a sole with splits, holes or different density materials
- it is heavy.

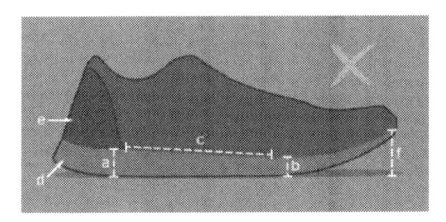

Illustration 51: Features of a bad shoe. a. An unnecessarily thick and soft sole at the rear of the shoe, b. An unnecessarily thick sole under the midfoot, c. Drop (slope from heel to toe), d. A flared heel, e. A stiff or angled heel counter, f. A turned-up toe box area.

How poor shoe choice affects your running and your body

In the previous illustrations (*50, 51*) shown above, we set out the good and bad features of shoes. We used *Illustration 50* to show the basic essentials of a running shoe; i.e. it needs to be thin, flat and flexible, and have good contact with the ground. However, there are also other things you should consider, such as making sure that the toe box doesn't squeeze your toes.

In *Illustration 51*, we pointed out the features of a shoe you should try to avoid. We now describe how these bad features will have a negative effect on your running, and potentially cause injury. We have firstly referred to them by the illustration number (*51*) and then by the corresponding letter in that illustration for your easy reference.

Sole thickness

Sole thickness includes zero-drop shoes and is shown in *Illustration 51.a* and *b*.

We have seen many ankle sprains that we attribute to thick-soled shoes, as thicker soles create instability and more stress up the body. If your shoes have thick soles, you will be unable to react to changing ground conditions and, because of this, you will increase your chances of ankle sprains and knee twists (see *Illustration 52*). Choosing shoes with a sole thickness between 5 mm and 10 mm is a good compromise between protection and performance. We give this range, as thickness depends on your skill level and the terrain. A better runner will manage a thinner shoe, and everyone will want a slightly thicker shoe on rough ground. Beware of 'trail' shoes, as they are usually too thick, stiff and heavy.

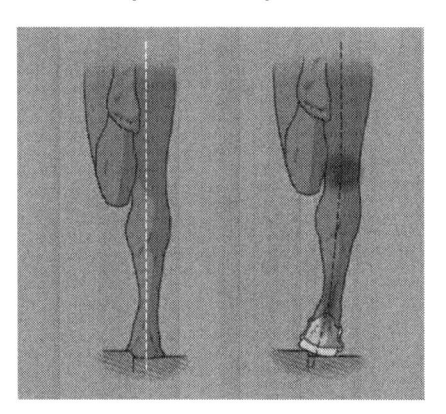

Illustration 52: Sole thickness. Compared to running barefoot (left figure), thick soles (right figure) reduce your ability to react to changing ground conditions. Thick soles increase the chances of ankle sprains (dark area) and knee twists (dark area) and create instability and more stress up the body.

Cushioning

Cushioning of the shoe is shown in *Illustration 51.a* and *b*.

Barefoot runners can run on hard smooth concrete with no problems since they do not strike the ground hard, demonstrating that impact is not an issue if you run well. Some cushioning is required for rough ground and over a longer distance, but ironically this makes you hit the ground harder.

Compared to a barefoot runner (*Illustration 53*, top figures), a runner wearing a soft-soled shoe (*Illustration 53*, bottom figures) needs to be on the ground longer (which also causes excessive pronation). This means, the shod runner must land sooner (leaning back, braking) and take off later (pushing forwards, accelerating). Therefore, cushioning increases your over-stride since your foot must land further in front of your hips to give your shoe time to squash under your weight. It makes you less stable, slower, it is harder work, and it is stressful, especially for Achilles tendons, the knees and the quads.

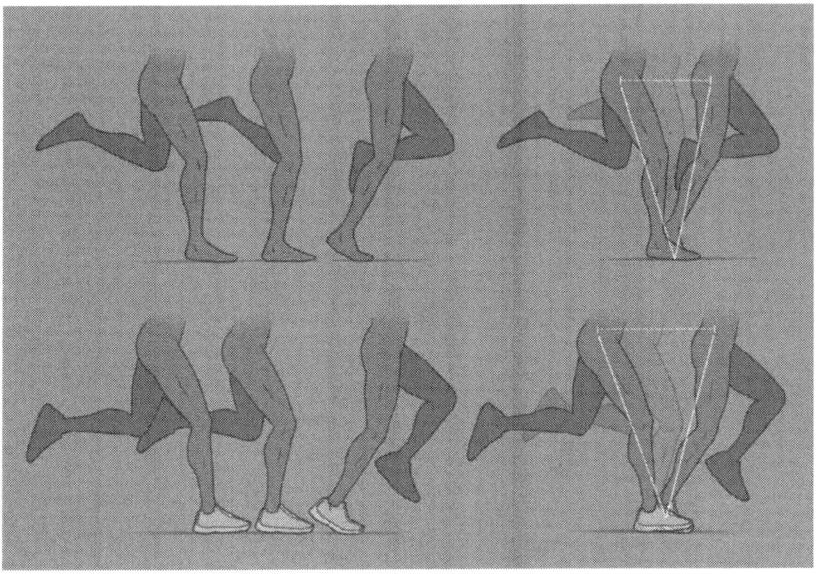

Illustration 53: Cushioning. Landing and take-off angles in a barefoot runner (top) and a runner wearing a soft-soled shoe (bottom) show how the shod runner needs to land leaning backwards (braking) and take-off more forwards, with more effort.

The drop

The drop of the shoe is shown in *Illustration 51.c* and is the slope from the heel to the forefoot. The drop is incorporated into most modern shoes, and yet it is the most damaging feature. The shoe industry 'standard' appears to be a 10–12 millimetre drop, but we see no reasonable argument for having any slope at all. As a matter of fact, as your running technique improves, you will become more and more aware of how shoes with angled soles negatively affect your running.

If your shoe has a drop, it is impossible to stand or to land with your body vertically aligned (OYF Rule #2). Perpetually standing on a sloped surface forces your spine out of alignment, which in turn weakens the postural muscles of your torso (see *Illustration 59*, Appendix B, *For podiatrists—treating runners*).

When running, you will tend to heel-strike—see Section 1.1, *Poor technique is mainly due to over-striding*—and when the sole is flat on the ground, you will be in a semi-squat position (see *Illustration 54*, bottom figures).

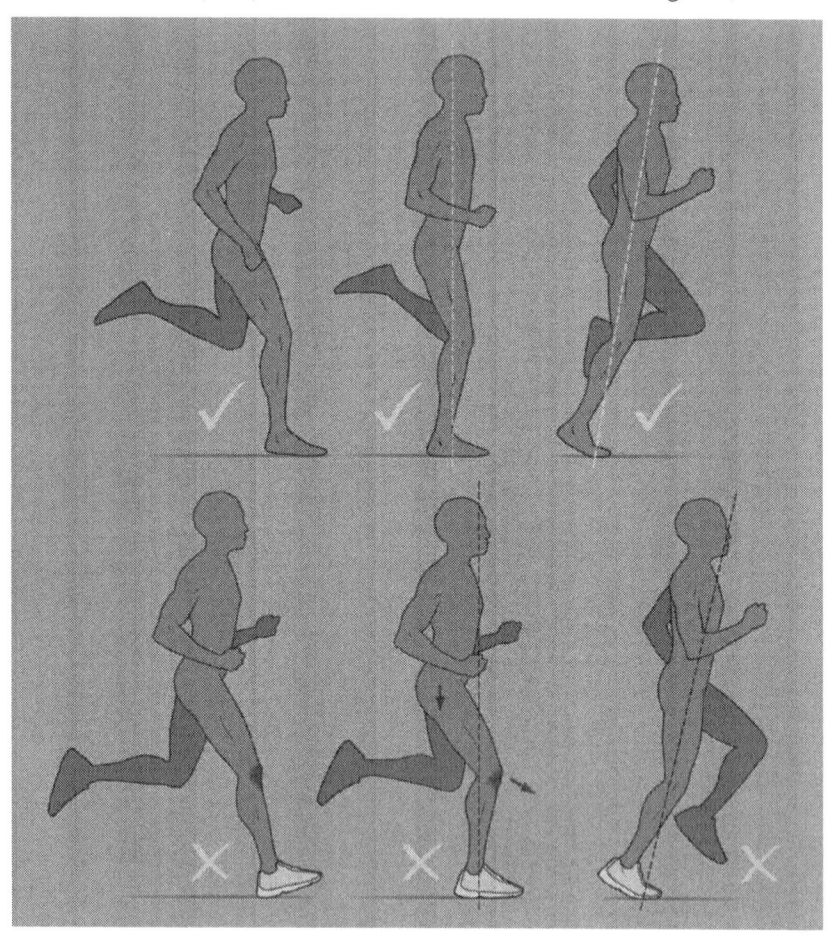

Illustration 54: The drop. Top. A barefoot runner. Bottom. If your shoe has a drop, it is impossible to land with your body vertically aligned (middle figure). The raised heel will force a change in technique, make you land your foot further in front of you or, at best, leave you with your knee pushed forwards and your hips dropping lower (arrows). This semi-squat position prevents you from getting a rebound and so requires you to push forwards into the next over-stride (right figure).

This means you will be over-striding; supporting your upper body more with your quads; and straining your knees, iliotibial bands and hip flexors. This poor technique also prevents your calves and your glutes from working properly, causing muscle imbalance and poor posture. Note that orthotics generally add 4 millimetres to the drop. Also, the smaller the shoe size, the steeper the slope.

Flared heel

In a shoe with a flared heel (*Illustration 51.d*), the back of the sole slopes outward. A heel that protrudes at the back makes a heel-strike more likely. It is of no use to a good runner and, like the stiff heel counter (*Illustration 51.e*), which was introduced to help the discredited heel–toe action, it should not be part of a shoe's construction.

Stiff or angled heel counter

A shoe with a stiff or angled heel counter is shown in *Illustration 51.e*.

The stiff heel counter is a relic of the days when heel-striking was advocated. It provided some stability for the backwards-leaning landings when using this stressful, damaging running action. Beware of heel counters that angle forwards as they can cut into your Achilles tendon.

Turned-up toe box

A shoe with a turned-up toe box area is shown in *Illustration 51.f*.

You rely on your toes for balance, whole-foot support and for pushing off during acceleration. Lifting your toes off the ground will mean a later, more forwards, more powerful take-off. Unless you are accelerating or going up hill, this more powerful take-off will be offset by an equivalent deceleration on landing, meaning you are working too hard.

All Heidi's patients that have presented with plantar fasciitis have been wearing shoes with raised heels and turned-up toes. A turned-up toe box, especially when combined with a raised heel, stresses the plantar fascia. It also opens up the metatarsal heads (ball of the foot) leaving them susceptible to metatarsalgia (see also Section 2.1, *Injuries to the feet*).

To test for plantar fasciitis, podiatrists stress the plantar fascia using the Windlass Test (pulling the toes up). As shown in *Illustration 55*, many shoes stress the foot this way all the time, even when standing.

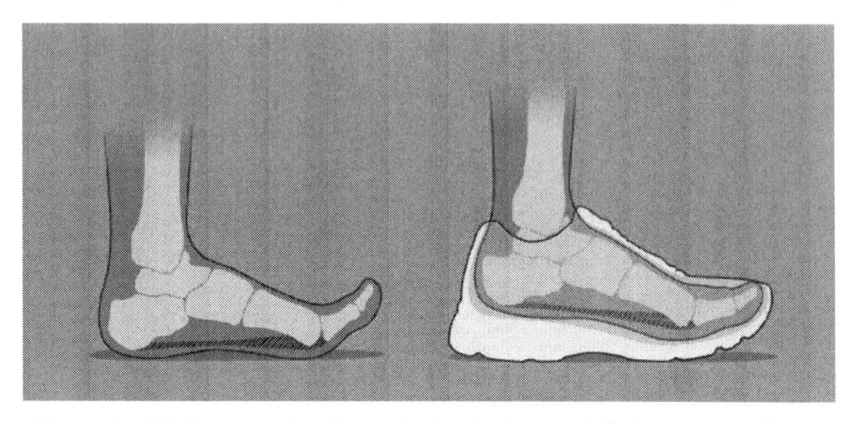

Illustration 55: Stress on the plantar fascia (dark area). Left. Stress caused by the Windlass Stress Test for plantar fasciitis. Right. The same stress caused by a chunky shoe with a turned-up toe box.

Sole stiffness

If your shoes have stiff soles, they will interfere with the natural roll of your foot as you land, and extra stress will be applied to areas such as the plantar fascia. Your foot should be allowed to follow its natural rolling action where it pronates, flexes and supinates—this is how your foot absorbs the impact and locks for that all important rebound.

Support, stability control

Many features of modern shoes are supposed to support your arches and control your landings in order to 'correct' over-pronation. This mechanical 'solution' will only lead to pain and injury, as it will force stress further up the body. As we have explained in Chapter 1, *How poor technique affects your running*, over-pronation is caused by over-striding, and if you fix over-striding, the over-pronation will stop (OYF Rule #3).

Narrow toe box

A narrow toe box squashes your toes and reduces your balance and control on landing. When people stop wearing shoes, their feet widen and this strongly suggests that shoes interfere with natural foot development. Squashing the forefoot can cause Morton's neuroma, which is a painful condition in the ball of the foot. It commonly occurs between the third and fourth toes, resulting in a sharp stinging, burning nerve pain or numbness.

Splits, holes, different density materials on the sole

Some shoes have holes to let water out (see *Illustration 56.1* and *56.2*). In our experience, these holes let water in through the soles, and they are stone-catchers. Holes in the forefoot area (*Illustration 56.1*) have caused toe fractures due to the middle part of a toe dropping into the hole.

Heidi has seen many patients with injuries that she thinks are caused by different density materials on the soles (*Illustration 56.3*). This is where the hard and soft parts make the shoe, in particular the heel, unstable. Such soles can cause partial dislocation (subluxation) of the cuboid (a cube-shaped bone on the outer side of the foot, approximately half-way between the heel and the forefoot), peroneal tendonitis or impingement of the medial plantar nerve. She thinks these different densities cause a whipping effect, as the foot ricochets between pronation and supination during the support phase of the landing.

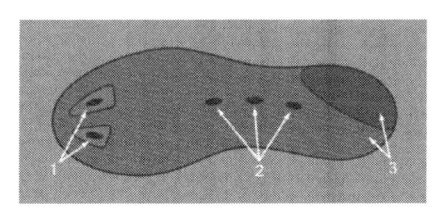

Illustration 56: *A shoe with holes in the forefoot area (1) and middle (2), and different density sole segments (3). If a shoe is thin enough there is no need to make it more flexible with slits or holes.*

Weight

There is never a need for a heavy shoe. There are two disadvantages to heavy shoes: they force you to either swing your legs or to lift your feet. Either of these will ruin your technique. In addition, a heavy shoe just wastes energy and over-uses your hip flexors. Your running action should be a natural, flowing motion.

14.3 Orthotics

Orthotics are artificial supports for the feet that compensate for a biomechanical abnormality. They are often unnecessarily prescribed for 'flat feet' or over-pronation, and negatively affect your running technique and your body in the same way as 'supportive' or raised-heel shoes (OYF Rule #2).

Although orthotics might provide temporary relief from pains and injuries, they are insidious in that they regularly cause more serious long-term problems. If you permanently use orthotics you have accepted that you have a lifelong deformity, which almost certainly is not the case.

Orthotics are bad for running technique because they:

- block pronation by tilting your foot in the opposite direction (they supinate the foot)
- reduce take-off power by raising your heel up in the shoe (typically 4 millimetres).

It is vital to have strength, flexibility and multi-directional movement throughout your feet and the lower legs. However, orthotics prevent this movement, inhibiting your ability to use the elastic energy through your feet and Achilles tendons to 'spring' off the ground, thus reducing your stride length. The only way to replace this lost stride length is to over-stride and to accept the injury risk associated with this. Your running times will also suffer due to the poor technique that orthotics promote.

Orthotics are bad for your body because they:

- can over-supinate the foot, which impinges the inside of the knee, which in turn stresses the medial meniscus and, at the same time, makes your landings harsh by removing pronation
- raise the heel (typically by 4 millimetres), which increases stress on the major joints; curves the spine; and stops the abdominals, gluteus medius and erector muscles functioning properly
- weaken the intrinsic muscles of the feet, which eventually leads to weakened postural muscles of the trunk (abdominal, erector spinae and gluteal muscles).

The adverse technique changes and the extra stresses that wearing orthotics cause are the major factors in the injuries that many of Heidi's patients present with. In the last decade (since 2006), Heidi has been able to rehabilitate all her patients' running injuries without using orthotics. For more information on how this is done, see Appendix B, *For podiatrists—treating runners*.

CHAPTER 15
HOW TO GET A HOT RUNNER'S BODY

Keith Bateman and Heidi Jones

While we were on our honeymoon at Waimea Bay, Hawaii, we were surprised and flattered to be approached by a father and daughter who had driven past us. They had seen us jogging back to our car in our swimmers and were intrigued. They approached us and said 'Excuse me, I hope you don't think this is weird, but how did you get bodies like that?' They themselves were in good shape and gym-goers. The daughter had said 'Dad, did you see that chick?' and the father replied 'No, I was checking out the guy!' We explained that we didn't go to the gym and we simply ran and that good running naturally produced a good body shape. We smiled all the way home.

We have often heard people say 'But you are lucky, you have a runner's body' or 'But you have good biomechanics'. Our flippant reply is usually 'Oh really! How did that happen?' Well, it happens naturally if you run well in the right shoes. The structure of your body changes according to the muscles you use. Not only will you get a good body shape from running well, running well can also help you overcome some physical disadvantages.

Even if you are 'unlucky' as in Heidi's case, where a family trait caused her right leg to be internally rotated such that it tended to clip the left leg when walking, you can still change for the better. During Heidi's transition to good running technique, from the 'classic' heel-striking that they had taught her at podiatry school, her right leg has straightened. Once she learnt to land consistently with her foot under her hips, her leg started adjusting! In her transition, she noticed that her right iliotibial band became tight; but in this case it was not from over-striding, but as a result of her leg settling back into its newly straightened position.

We have seen this type of re-alignment happen even with runners who have weak glutes and wobble like a baby giraffe. After a technique change, the glutes strengthen and the wayward legs become aligned, as do outward-facing feet. So do not worry about your current shape: run well, and your shape will improve along with your technique. Take a photo now, and again in six months; you will be amazed at the transformation that good running technique can bring about.

15.1 Body strength through running

If you run with good technique, keep to a sensible running program, and wear the correct shoes, you will automatically build the right muscles and attain the right body shape. On the other hand, if you sit around all day, your hamstrings and glutes will gradually weaken. If your foot lands considerably in front of your hips, your quads and glutes will be out of balance. If you encase your feet in brick-like shoes or use orthotics, your feet will not strengthen and your abdominals and butt will weaken. It's as simple as that!

Strength for running should come from running. Even when walking, if you are near-vertically aligned whenever your foot is supporting you, then your body will strengthen and change from your toes to your head (OYF Rule #2).

15.2 Things you don't need to worry about

Cross-training (training in a sport other than running) is good for all-round fitness, but is not necessary for running strength. However, it is a useful aid for avid runners who are injured and need to be active. Other activities like walking and swimming can also aid recovery by increasing blood flow without stress.

This leads to our tenth OYF Rule.

> **OYF Rule #10: Drills and exercises should directly relate to the running action**
>
> If you are trying to strengthen or rehabilitate after injury, then the most useful drills and exercises are those that most closely resemble the running action—many do not. For instance, glute-strengthening exercises should be done on one leg, in a standing position. Otherwise you are not being specific enough for strengthening the muscles you need for running. Use drills where you can land whole-foot as much as possible and don't skid when you land.

Lunges and anything more than a quarter knee squat can easily put excessive pressure on your knee joint and are a fast-track way of wearing it out. We do not regard them to be related to a good running action. At no time do you need to do anything similar to a lunge or a squat during a run, except perhaps if you need to go to the toilet! Exercise is specific to what you do (OYF Rule#10). To be a fast runner, you have to practice running fast. Running with good form will help you to achieve this. Doing squats will help you to be good at doing squats!

Stair running is not helpful for running, unless you are training for a stair running race. Running stairs forces you into an artificial stride pattern. The set height and width of the stairs is unlikely to match the stride length you need for the speed you are running at. It is likely that you will be forced into over-striding and excessive quad use. You are much better off finding a hill, where you can control the take-off angle, power and cadence and maintain some speed and good form (OYF Rule#10).

Flat feet are generally not a hindrance, especially if there are no arthritic changes or joint deformities. Many great runners have flat feet. With the correct landing, the whole foot pronates and therefore arch height does not need to be taken into account. Additionally, running with good form with light shoes actually strengthens the arches. Both our foot arches have become higher, stronger and springier due to technique changes and by removing supportive shoes.

Having 'duck feet' (feet pointing outwards) does not hinder good running. We have independently arrived at the conclusion that this is most often associated with a muscle imbalance in runners who over-stride and consequently under-use their glutes. As long as there are no associated foot deformities, this alignment of the feet can be changed over time with the introduction of glute-strengthening exercises, good running technique and consciously pointing your feet forwards.

Having 'baby giraffe syndrome' does not prevent good running. We have had a number of cases of young teenagers with flat feet, knock knees, feet pointing outwards like a duck, very weak glute muscles, and who walk and run like a newly-born baby giraffe. Those teenagers who have been put into light shoes and taught to run well have become good runners with a strong body and no pain. However, where the parents have insisted on retaining chunky shoes and orthotics, the teenagers remain weak, suffer years of pain and finally give up running altogether. It could have been so different!

Asymmetry is normal. People generally think that everyone is 100% symmetrical, or should be; however, in reality it is common for people to have feet that are different in size or shape, or have legs that differ in length.

Leg length difference might seem like a hindrance, but is not necessarily so. Having legs of different length is very noticeable when standing or walking, but when you are running well a minor leg length difference hardly matters. This is because, if you run well, your landings are separated by the flight phase and are independent of each other. Your muscles, tendons and ligaments are able to work together to adjust the flex independently for each leg. A leg length difference therefore should not cause extra stress at the hips, unless you are over-striding.

If you were born with a leg length difference (and many people are), your body will have adapted to it, probably by dropping one hip and curving your spine, and this will be normal for you. We believe a 2 centimetre difference is manageable without artificial aids. Therefore, unless you have acquired a leg length difference through an accident or surgery, we suggest you sort your running technique first and then, if you still have pain, seek medical advice. Building up one shoe will render skilful running impossible and increase the possibility of injury.

15.3 How do you spot a good runner?

The great news about running with good form is that you don't need to worry about your body shape. You'll get thousands of whole-body strengthening and body-reshaping steps every time you go out for a run. Rolling out tight muscles and going through stretching routines will no longer be necessary and running pains will largely be a thing of the past.

Good running produces a good body shape; note the characteristic features whereby you can recognise a good runner in *Illustration 57*:

- A tight butt from working the glutes every landing (*Illustration 57.1*). Poorer runners will have developed their quadriceps at the expense of their glutes.
- Strong, 'cut' hamstrings and calf muscles for the same reason (*Illustration 57.2*). Poorer runners have less-developed muscles at the back of their legs.
- Core strength, not from gym work but by simply landing vertically aligned and naturally, using the core muscles to stabilise the torso (*Illustration 57.3*). Poorer runners have to do core-strengthening work on top of their running (OYF Rule #2).
- Light shoes (*Illustration 57.4*). Poorer runners can usually be seen wearing chunky shoes.

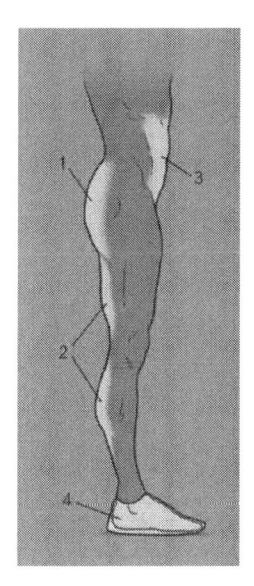

Illustration 57: Good running produces a good body shape. The characteristics whereby you can recognise a good runner: 1. A tight butt, 2. Strong, 'cut' hamstrings and calf muscles, 3. Core strength. 4. Light shoes.

Heidi says: you can't fake it!

I can tell a good runner just by their physique. Generally, their body will be tight: they will have a firm bum, hamstrings and calf muscles. When I was single and working at St Vincent's Hospital, one of the orthopaedic surgeons introduced his young registrar as a runner. His physique didn't indicate this, and without saying a word I looked at the registrar, reached around and felt his hamstrings, looked at them both and said 'No. He's not!' The registrar laughed and said 'Well, actually, you're right. I am a cyclist.' I don't think he minded being corrected as he had enjoyed the examination.

Looks can be deceiving …

Take a look at *Illustration 58*, which has been adapted from an actual photo of a young female runner. At first glance, this runner has a great body shape. However, when we look in more detail, we see a big curvature in the spine. She is standing and landing misaligned (see OYF Rule #2) and wearing chunky shoes. Her over-striding has produced strong quads and weak glutes, which in turn have changed her body shape by adjusting her hip position. The over-striding is confirmed by the toe-running, the chunky shoes and the unbalanced landing.

If you draw a vertical line through the ground-contact point (which is only the forefoot in this case), you will see how she is sitting back (most of her body is behind her foot). The bad news is that this runner is likely to encounter pain in the forefoot, Achilles tendon, ankle, knee, back and neck. The good news is that change is easy and, although it will be years before her body shape becomes what it should be, it will be a pleasant and fruitful journey should she wish to take it.

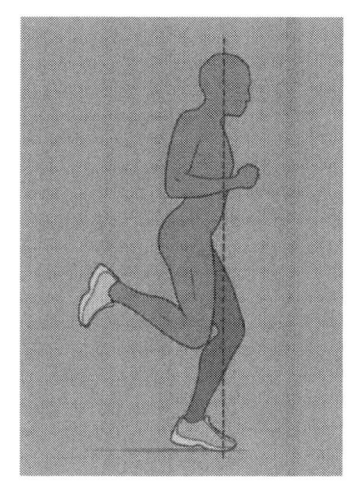

Illustration 58: Adapted from a photo of a young female runner. Poor running in chunky shoes produces a poor body shape: weak glutes, strong quads and a significant curve in the lower back. The vertical line through the ground-contact point shows most of her body is behind her foot.

CHAPTER 16
TIPS AND TRAPS

Keith Bateman and Heidi Jones

In this chapter, we offer a range of tips covering body care, training and racing, and we advise you of the many traps that runners fall into.

16.1 General training tips

Take care not to get sidetracked by advertising and fads (remember, we consider most shoes to be fads). For your normal running, you can forget about your VO2 Max, smart watches, heart rate monitors, special diets, vitamins, running 'junk miles', compression tights, weights, and so on. Leave these distractions until you are running well and you will probably find you don't need most of them after all.

Do not attempt to run through pain, injury or sickness. Rest is our personal choice in these circumstances. There is always another race. Do not mask pain with anti-inflammatories. Pain means there is a problem and the inflammation is a necessary part of the healing process. You can easily end up with a stress fracture if you mask pain.

Make technique the most important part of your running, from which everything else develops. Learn to run with good form over a short distance and then gradually extend the distance. Long races might be fashionable, but you won't learn to run well doing them. So, don't go beyond your range—the range at which your feet and calf muscles are too tired to work properly. Why practice running badly? It is possible to run very fast times on relatively small amounts of training if your technique is good, since every landing is building muscle in the right places.

Gradually increase your distance until you can run the race distance with good form. Start with 3-kilometre or 5-kilometre races and run them well. Running 'junk miles' simply gets you better at running badly, and causes injury. You do need to stress yourself in training with speed work and long runs to improve, but we suggest this should be left until you are running well.

After running, you should feel no pain, as if you have been for a swim. And any muscle soreness from overdoing it should disappear quickly.

If your running friends start off fast on the warm-up, start ten minutes earlier so you can warm up your muscles. Always start slowly and gradually build up speed. If you run fast without warm, reactive muscles you will over-stride; see 'Spring, don't swing' (OYF Rule #5).

Try not to run on long sections of cambered surfaces, such as sloping beaches or roads. This will cause extra stress on one leg and hip.

When you look at faster runners, don't see them as being special in biomechanics, posture or strength; just see them as being further advanced in their training. When you run well, you too will acquire these attributes and people will look at you in the same way! Until you have all elements of your running in place, you don't know how good you can be.

16.2 'I am different', 'I can't run because ...'

No, you are not different. Even runners with 'bad knees', 'bad backs', and so on, can change their technique and help their body to repair by running efficiently. Nobody has perfect biomechanics—different size feet, high arches, flat feet, different leg lengths, etcetera, are normal. Asymmetry is normal. And your body will have adapted to accommodate these idiosyncrasies, by changing its structure, and the strength of muscles, tendons, ligaments and bones. Your body will continue to adapt, which is why your technique improvement will continue for many years (See Chapter 15, *How to get a hot runner's body*).

For two people running efficiently, the only real differences are the strength-to-weight ratio (how easily they get off the ground), fitness, endurance, and race tactics. Being overweight or older will also be a disadvantage, but if you run well you will be able to train more, and you will be able to reach your potential.

16.3 Care for your body

Drink water after a run, whether you feel like it or not. If you feel lethargic, before you reach for the quick-fix chocolate bar, check your urine. If it's dark in colour, then you might be tired from dehydration. On the other hand, don't drink excessive amounts of water in the lead-up to races, as this can wash the sodium out of your system (hyponatremia), which will give you a serious headache, and can be very dangerous.

If you get headaches after your runs, make sure you are not lacking in salts. However, don't immediately resort to so-called sports drinks. Sports drinks can be good for specific situations, such as when doing a marathon or if you are doing heavy lifting work all day in summer, but they are unnecessary on a daily basis. They are generally high in sugar too, so ask your dentist what damage they might do to your teeth! In most cases, you can use water and salty foods to restore your body's natural balance. Sports drinks mainly replace lost carbohydrates and electrolytes, and don't usually have the necessary nutrients for muscles to regenerate themselves. Milk is a good alternative.

Don't be fooled into unnecessarily taking supplements and vitamins. You should only need these if you are recovering from illness or when these have been prescribed for a specific condition. It's better to get the nutrients you need by eating a wide range of fruits and especially vegetables.

If you suffer from athlete's foot or itchy feet, apply rubbing alcohol on the affected area. We keep a spray bottle of this in the bathroom for spraying between our toes after showering.

If you have hard skin or you feel heat or get blisters in certain areas, look for the cause in this order:

> 1. Are your shoes too small, either in length, or more commonly, in width?
>
> 2. Are orthotics causing pressure that is redistributed to the area where you get blisters?
>
> 3. Are your feet moving in your shoes due to the stop–start effect (see Section 2.2, *Injuries to the rest of the body*) caused by poor running technique?

The cause of your foot problem could be a mixture of all of these, but getting your feet back into good shape over the next few years is simple: all can be changed with a little effort and time to adjust.

16.4 Racing

If going for a personal best time, run the first 90% of the race at your previous best pace; this way you will be certain that it is not too fast. The last 10% will look after itself.

Do not relax near the finish line: always assume someone is chasing you down! Make the last 200 metres your fastest. Don't look behind or you will give those behind you renewed confidence.

Feeling bad in a race? Remember the runner next to you feels as bad as you do, but you are stronger willed. And remember that you have always felt worse in training and that you got through it in training, so you can now.

Tell yourself you only feel bad because you are going fast, not because you are doing badly. Remind yourself that giving up wastes all the good work you have invested getting to this point in the race, and if you give up now you'll have to do it all again for that best-ever time!

If you are working your way through the field, rest behind the runner(s) in front before making a move, as you have used extra energy catching them. When you pass them, do it decisively. Go, count to 50, and don't look back.

In track races, run close to the inside of the lane when you can. The 400-metre line is measured 20 centimetres from the inner edge, or 30 centimetres if there is a barrier. Running in lane two is 7 metres longer per lap. Be careful, though, not to step on the edge of the track when you are tired.

In road races, remember that the course is measured along the shortest possible route that you can run within the course limits. To ensure that you run the shortest distance, look ahead and run a straight line where you can, rather than following the curves of the road. This will gain you some valuable metres and you will also find it psychologically beneficial.

For long races on hot days, try putting vaseline on your eyebrows to keep the sweat from your forehead out of your eyes.

For men, in longer races, or if your running top material is a little rough, consider covering your nipples with bandaids or tape. It could save a lot of soreness and blood loss!

People frequently overlook the simple action of correctly tying up their shoes, tying them either too loose or too tight. It's surprising how many people have to stop to re-tie their laces, losing valuable time in the process, and how many end the race with pain on the top of their foot because they are tied too tight.

And finally, don't try anything new for a race: no new diet, no new clothes, and *definitely* no new shoes. Thoroughly trial everything you are going to eat or wear in the weeks before a race.

16.5 Trails

Running trails is no different to running on roads, except that you might need a slightly thicker sole as protection from stones. However, if you run well, there is little impact and you will be faster in a thin shoe and have less chance of turning an ankle.

On downhill sections, you might come across raised-earth bars, designed to force water off the path to reduce erosion. Try to time your take-off before these so you fly over them and continue running the same gradient rather than interrupting your flow by landing on, and leaping off, the bar.

Where there is a sharp turn and the slope falls away from you, to avoid sliding, take the corner wide so you can run around the bank, if there is one. Your feet will land flat against the 'wall', like a cyclist at a velodrome or a slalom skier using ruts, and you won't slip sideways.

16.6 Don't neglect side-view video reviews

We mean to nag you because improving your technique is a brain-changing exercise, and to improve you need to continually review what you are actually doing, not what you think you are doing. Therefore, don't neglect a side-view video (OYF Rule #1) and study the individual frames of your landings to see what's really happening.

Examples of deceptive images:
- High-speed camera shots of airborne runners can be misleading. Guessing where and how their foot will land is problematic. It depends on their speed and how high off the ground they are. You cannot determine these factors from a still photograph. The only way to properly check your landing is when the whole foot is on the ground.
- A good runner moving at high speed gets 'stretched out': their foot gets left a long way behind their hips. Single-frame images of the stretched-out back leg just after the take-off appear to show the runner driving forwards. However, they are not driving forwards—their foot has simply been left behind (OYF Rule #7).

16.7 Don't force changes to your cadence

The two most common misconceptions about cadence are that you need to do more steps and shorter strides to reduce your over-stride, and that you need to try to run at a set cadence of around 180 steps per minute.

Rather than focusing on your cadence, you should be looking at improving your technique to eventually give you more time in the air, a naturally longer stride, and a naturally correct cadence (OYF Rule #8).

Misconception 1: you can reduce over-striding with more steps and shorter strides

This misconception is based on walking—where one foot is always on the ground—not running, where there is a flight phase that varies with speed.

If you are already over-striding, then doing more steps will simply mean that you end up doing lots of smaller, faster over-strides. You will end up with a shorter stride length; but, in order to improve your times, you would have to set an impossibly fast cadence.

For example, take the case of a runner who is currently over-striding. For a beginner, they would typically be running at 6 minutes per kilometre (1000 metres), with 165 steps per minute, so that their stride length will be 1.01 metre, as this calculation shows:

$$1000 \text{ m} / (165 \times 6) = 1.01 \text{ m}$$

Increasing their cadence to 180 steps per minute at the same speed would result in a stride length of 0.93 metre:

$$1000 \text{ m} / (180 \times 6) = 0.93 \text{ m}$$

As you can see from the above figures, with a cadence of 180, they have managed to reduce their stride length by about 8 centimetres, but they still have a problem. If they want to achieve a reasonable running speed of say 5 minutes per kilometre, with that same stride length, their cadence will have to increase to 215 steps per minute, as shown below:

$$1000 \text{ m} / (215 \times 5) = 0.93 \text{ m}$$

This is very hard work and cannot be sustained.

Misconception 2: you need to try to run at a set cadence of around 180 steps per minute

Don't try to be a metronome!

It is quite often voiced that the ideal to be reached is a set cadence of 180 steps per minute, since this is the bottom end of the range at which a good runner would normally run. This was initially developed by researchers who studied elite runners and has been passed on by coaches and running groups. However, individuals will peak at different cadences and there are all sorts of factors that come into play. In other words, 180 steps per minute is an arbitrary figure and, as mentioned above, cadence should come naturally.

By all means, measure your cadence indirectly with a smart watch or by video, but check it after your run. Use your cadence as a guide to how well you are running, but don't change your running to try to achieve a set cadence. Getting fixated on cadence or using a metronome just helps you to count 180+ bad steps. Learn to land balanced and everything else will adjust naturally around this, including your cadence.

A balanced landing is how to find your right cadence

The key to reduce an over-stride and increase speed is a balanced landing. This will enable a springy take-off, giving you more airtime, a longer stride and also a higher cadence. This is how to reduce your over-stride while increasing your stride length, and how to go a lot faster in the process. See OYF Rule #4.

16.8 Don't sweat about your 'vertical oscillation'

As you saw in *Good and bad technique on the treadmill* in Chapter 10, when you run well, you will be going mostly up and down. This is 'good' vertical oscillation, which is largely produced by using the elasticity of your body from landing near to vertically aligned. If you over-stride, there will be more horizontal, forwards and backwards movement along the treadmill, but there will also be up and down movement. However, in this case it is 'bad' vertical oscillation because it is as a result of you braking and collapsing at the waist upon landing, and then having to push upwards and forwards at each take-off in order to regain lost speed. Therefore, vertical oscillation, just like cadence, is an indicator, but not a good measure of, efficiency in running.

Some people actually advocate keeping the hips parallel with the ground (zero 'vertical oscillation' as some say), but this is impossible, as your hips must leave the ground to run. Don't try this, as it means the only way you can move or keep moving is to lift or swing your foot in front of you; that is, by over-striding.

16.9 Don't change your foot strike

Changing your foot-landing angle will not stop your foot landing in front of you. Don't try to forefoot-strike or midfoot-strike (see also Section 1.1, *Poor technique is mainly due to over-striding*), or you will indeed be 'striking' the ground instead of achieving a balanced, progressive, smooth landing that will serve you well for the rest of your (extended) running life. Be especially careful not to change from heel-striking to forefoot running, as injury is almost assured. The only time your forefoot should be taking extra load is when running up hill or accelerating.

Our advice also applies to the whole-foot, under-the-hips landing that we describe throughout this book. Monitoring your landings provides excellent feedback, but the perfectly balanced landing that you seek will only come by balancing your whole body.

16.10 Don't try to 'fall forwards'

Some people have been told that they should constantly fall when running and that gravity provides a proportion of the forwards motion when running. However, this idea runs against the physical laws of motion. Gravity pulls you down, not forwards—you go forwards mostly because you are already going forwards, rather like freewheeling on a bicycle—and your speed is reduced by braking and increased by pushing.

Assuming that you start and finish your run standing, the total of your forwards 'falling' must equal the total amount of your backwards-leaning braking. This means that, at constant speed, the more forwards your take-off, the more you are leaning back, braking when you land. Therefore, if you constantly tilt forwards and you are not accelerating, you must be over-striding.

16.11 Don't just copy others

Do not try to copy what you think you see others doing. Remember, you cannot perfect your running technique by watching others. You have to develop your own good technique and you will do this by following Keith's Lessons (Chapters 5 to 10).

16.12 Don't be conned into setting the wrong goals

Common phrases seen on television, on tee-shirts and in publications will encourage you to 'never give up', to 'dig deep', to think 'no pain, no gain'. If you follow these ideas, it is extremely doubtful that you will remain uninjured long enough to become a good, fast runner. Pushing yourself to endure pain is a high-risk, inefficient strategy, which we are convinced leads to skeletal damage. Technique first, strength and speed will follow.

We see many injured runners whose goal has been to complete a marathon or half marathon, or even a 10-kilometre race, but who haven't considered how they are running. While such race goals are admirable, if you want to run well into your older years, then your goal should be to learn to run well with no pain. If you learn the technique of good running and let your muscles and skills build, you will become faster and stronger. You will then surprise yourself: you will far exceed what would have been your goals.

Become a thinking runner: more skill, less effort.

16.13 Don't be swayed by sales gimmicks

Sales people routinely use machines and other technology to measure your foot 'type' or running action, but what they measure is irrelevant to choosing the right shoe. If they assess or video you from behind, they don't understand running biomechanics and will give you the wrong advice. We often see slow, injured runners in new chunky shoes who say things like 'But I went to a well-respected running shop …', 'But they analysed my running gait …', 'But they put me on a machine and identified my foot type …', 'But they said I over-pronate …', 'But …'.

Sales staff will play on your fear of injury, your desire for speed, and even say that you have a problem with your biomechanics. They will make unsupported, unscientific claims and present this nonsense as fact. They will talk to you with confidence, telling you about foot strike, supination, pronation, or cushioning for impact protection; but we say they do not understand the physics of running. Most of the shop staff probably believe what they are saying, but these distractions lead you to assume that your running gait determines a shoe 'type'; that over-pronation is a physical, not a technique problem; that a certain foot 'type' requires a certain type of shoe. We see no evidence to support these ideas. They are smoke screens to help sell you shoes that you don't need.

We hope you will see through these clever sales tricks and find the shoe that will help you to run your best. When you reach the final stage of precision in your running, you will realise that you would not have made it without the correct shoes.

Test before you buy

Once you have found a good shoe, try to do a test run. If the shop allows you to take them outside that's ideal. If there is a treadmill in the shop, use that. Otherwise, the exercises in Chapter 5, *Lesson One: Landing*, are a good test: bounce up and down in bare feet and then in the shoes. You should still feel bouncy with the shoes on.

When you replace your shoes with the same model, make sure you check for 'upgrades'. Shoe manufacturers often keep the same name for the shoe but change the design, usually adding a detrimental feature such as arch support or a section with different density materials on the sole.

16.14 Where you might go wrong

Here we summarise all the ways you can go wrong when running:

- trying to land on a specific part of your foot (you should adjust your overall balance instead)
- decreasing your stride length to reduce your over-stride*
- increasing your stride length by stretching out (think about how a kangaroo increases its stride length: it doesn't reach out in front of itself)
- constantly leaning forwards and kicking your feet up behind you
- lifting your knees**
- lifting your feet in front of you
- trying to reduce your time on the ground (this will happen naturally when you land balanced)
- trying to keep the trajectory of your hips parallel with the ground
- pumping your arms
- wearing a zero-drop shoe that has more than a 10 millimetre sole thickness.

* Decreasing your stride length works for walking, but it is not good practice for running. It does not account for a flight phase and it does not improve technique. It simply makes you do more, smaller over-strides. Runners with good technique generally have a higher natural cadence because their balanced landings mean they can take off without delay. Swinging your legs to get a higher cadence doesn't make you a good runner.

** Lifting your knees will give you tight hip flexors and should not be part of your running. With good technique, your knees will naturally rise with the rest of your body. They will rise more at higher speeds and during accelerations. Raising your knees artificially will slow you down and reduce your take-off power because you need to lean back to do it.

APPENDIX A
FOR COACHES—APPLYING THE LESSONS

Keith Bateman

This appendix is written specifically for coaches. In it, I show you how to introduce OYF Running and my system of technique change into your coaching sessions. I emphasise the message that you need to get across to your clients, and describe the theory that I always explain to my clients before I start them on any of the exercises. I then go through the main points of each lesson, from Chapter 5 to Chapter 10, before finishing off with some post-session tips.

I have been coaching athletes for over 40 years. I started out by teaching skiing when I was 19, and my desire to do cross-country skiing in 1989 got me into running. I emigrated to Australia in 2000, at the age of 45, and joined an elite running group in Sydney, conducted by Sean Williams. I learnt a lot from this group but, even though my race times were decent, I couldn't improve beyond a certain point.

My own interest in biomechanics led me to get assessed, but the over-emphasis on detailed measurements and strengthening exercises recommended in the biomechanical assessment report, made me question the focus of their analysis. I buckled down to conduct my own analysis of what was going on, and I was rewarded with an insight into what was holding me back in 2007. My running technique was all wrong! From that moment on, I saw clearly that poor technique was the key problem, and I was able to go on and develop my own system for correcting running technique.

After meeting Heidi, I found that her specific and well-researched exercises rounded out my own system. We now had a complete guide

(Keith's Lessons) to transitioning into good form, a set of strengthening exercises (Heidi's Strengthening Program), and a set of specific rehabilitation exercises (Chapter 13) in the case of an injury. We formalised our knowledge of good technique and the correct way of running in 2014, when we introduced OYF Running in the first edition of this book.

A.1 Preparation for technique change

Before you introduce clients to the OYF Running technique changes, you will need to tell them that they will have to cut back their training. You will probably find, as I do, that they are used to running long distances and training hard, and that they are reluctant to cut back. You need to impress on them that, as they change their technique, they have to allow time for their body to adjust: previously underused muscles and tendons will be doing much more work. Building up the necessary muscular infrastructure can take up to 12 months. Heidi and I offer guidance on the transition in Chapter 12, *Managing your transition*, and this information should be given to all your clients and understood before you change their technique. Ideally, every client will have read this book and have started Heidi's Strengthening Program before their first session with you.

Your clients must be fully aware that they need to cut back to as little as 2 kilometres per run, two or three times per week, and to rebuild from there. They will not be able to resume 'full' training for many months and they certainly cannot race. This rule applies to everyone, even the best runners. I had one client who was already running 30 minutes for 10 kilometres and both he and his coach thought a technique session with me within 5 weeks of his next race would be fine. It wasn't! The client said that by 6 kilometres he thought his calf muscles were 'about to explode'. He was lucky to finish and not be out of action for weeks.

Although your clients might complain about the changes to their normal training routine, the upside is that after the transition period they will run much faster with less effort and will be far less likely to have a significant injury, which means they should be able to train consistently in the future.

A.2 My coaching sessions—overview

All my coaching sessions are the same and they are reproduced in the lessons in this book. A typical first session covers lessons one to five (except hills) and one or two exercises from Lesson Six. The first session lasts between an hour and 90 minutes, depending on the number of clients and how quickly they adopt the techniques. In subsequent sessions, I review the same lessons and introduce more refinement exercises from Lesson Six, plus hill running from Lesson Five.

I find it is important to get across the main points of good technique before we start training. I know this is probably not what you would normally do, but it is important to change their way of thinking from the outset. Clients who come to my sessions and have read the book beforehand usually perform much better with their re-training, as they already understand the concepts.

When I start the actual exercises, I tailor my sessions to individual clients' needs: I don't do all of the exercises with everyone and I sometimes need to spend longer on an exercise with some of them. However, all the exercises have the same purpose: to achieve a balanced landing. Therefore, if an exercise doesn't work, I will skip it and try an alternative. After my sessions, I review—together with my clients—the areas they need to work on, and I keep in touch with them to help them continue with Keith's Lessons. I continue to provide follow-up support via email and social media.

A.3 My coaching sessions—details

In my private coaching sessions, I use videos to show the client's technique improvement. I explain this in detail in A.6, *General tips*, at the end of this appendix. Here, I explain how my group sessions usually unfold.

The theory

I start my group sessions with a theoretical part in which I explain the following elements step by step.

Landing and the consequences: there's only one problem

I first explain that the central problem for all runners is over-striding, which I define as landing with the foot in front of the hips. Over-striding will cause runners to lean back, even after they have fully landed. I point out how the force of impact on landing is excessive because runners are pushing against their direction of travel, and that the faster they run, the worse it gets. I then list the types of injuries this causes, such as shin splints, knee injuries, iliotibial band problems, hip flexor pain, back pain and neck pain. These injuries are discussed in more detail in Chapter 2, *Poor technique causes injuries*.

Getting a 'good' stride length

Next, I tell my clients how good runners get a much longer and more efficient stride length by flying rather than walking along the ground. I find a good way to demonstrate this is by using the treadmill comparison (see *Good and bad technique on the treadmill* in Chapter 10). To show how it is possible to get this long stride with minimum effort, I get my clients to measure my stride length as I run past them at an easy pace. I count my landings, 'one, two, one, two,' and I ask them to place my discarded shoes on the ground to mark two of my consecutive landing points.

I am frequently asked to repeat the exercise, as they are amazed that I can have a stride length as big as 1.25 metres without stretching out my legs. I explain that it is my speed and my height off the ground that gives me that almost effortless long stride. This drives home the point that with application and attention to good technique, they too will be able to 'bounce and fly' (OYF Rule #4).

Getting airborne by landing vertically aligned

Once clients understand the difference between a good stride length and a bad stride length, they are ready to learn about how to get a good spring off the ground. I explain that a good runner lands with the body near-vertically aligned, which allows the runner to rebound off the ground with little wasted energy and a minimum of pushing. This 'bounce' is not visible in itself, but is incorporated in the take-off, and the instant the runner achieves this level of skill, it results in a sudden increase in stride length and speed. I regularly witness a dramatic increase in speed of 15% once clients get this right.

In this book (Section 3.2, *Take-off*), I describe two ways to leave the ground: the 'bounce' and the 'push'. Better runners will have more bounce because they land more vertically aligned and a large part of their take-off power comes from the elasticity in their legs that this balanced landing gives them. On the other hand, poorer runners will land leaning back and have little or no 'bounce' potential, and so they push forwards to regain lost speed. This is demonstrated in the *Beach check* in Section 10.2, *Other checks and exercises to refine your form*.

Using the feet and legs as springs

After explaining the need for a vertical landing to my clients, it is time to give them a little more detail about how landing vertically aligned produces take-off power through stored energy in the foot and Achilles tendon. I go through how the foot pronates upon contact with the ground, explaining that the full load of the landing takes place once the foot is under the hips, and how the foot locks into a supinated position again for a strong take-off.

I then move on to the elasticity of the calf and Achilles tendon, explaining how these extend as the heel touches the ground, and then how these retract. I stress that when extension–retraction is combined with the foot action, the runner experiences a good 'spring' off the ground.

Shoes and orthotics

The clients now understand how the combination of landing balanced and the mechanisms of the foot, calf and Achilles tendon work together to produce an efficient take-off. This means they are ready to hear how shoes and orthotics interfere with landing and take-off, which is an important defence against the conflicting information they will likely receive when buying shoes.

Heidi's podiatry skills have been invaluable in detailing the following problems:

- An arch support or orthotics in a shoe takes away the elastic capacity of the foot to absorb and provide lift. In short, orthotics restrict pronation.
- A shoe with a drop will stop the Achilles tendon and calf muscle fully stretching, and will leave the runner in a semi-squat position. This means less take-off 'spring', which leaves 'driving' forwards and over-striding as the only alternative for the runner to maintain speed.
- A cushioned shoe leads to greater time on the ground. This is because it takes time for the cushioning in the shoe to compress. This increase in time on the ground can only be achieved by landing with the foot further in front (over-striding). There is also the danger of ankle twists and tendon tears, which frequently occur in shoes that have thick or stiff soles. You will find a more detailed analysis in Chapter 14, *Shoes—what you need to know*.

This is the end of the theoretical part of my session.

The activities

The first practical thing I get my clients to do is take off their shoes. Removing shoes allows everyone to land well, and to feel what a good landing is like. This is a very important part of the lessons. Barefoot on flat grass is the best surface for my lessons. If you are unable to get the class to go barefoot due to outdoor conditions, then sports halls and running tracks are highly suitable; even smooth concrete paths work well. If the client objects to running barefoot, then the lightest shoes possible (thin, flat and flexible) should be suggested.

The first three lessons (Chapters 5 to 7) are conducted in a small area and last about 10 minutes in total. These three lessons show the clients how to land, start and accelerate. Next, we practise Keith's Game Changer (Chapter 8) five or six times, and then we move on to exercises the clients can use in their everyday runs. Here, clients learn the standard starting method described in Chapter 9, followed by a selection of exercises from Chapter 10. At the end of the session, clients should be confident in knowing when their technique is failing and be familiar with the methods of self-correction.

Having detailed what goes on in my sessions, I now highlight the aspects of good technique that we are trying to get across to the clients at each point.

Lesson One—Landing

The landing lesson (Chapter 5) is vital to your clients' progress because they need to know what a whole-foot, vertically-aligned landing feels like to successfully work through the other lessons. The good news is that your clients will find these exercises (EXERCISE 5.1, 5.2 and 5.3) easy to do.

There are, however, a few things you need to be sure to mention:

- The heel must make solid contact with the ground; this will feel strange to them if they have been wearing shoes with a drop.
- The landings will be much harder than expected while stationary and when moving slowly.
- The firmness of the landings will decrease with speed and will hardly be noticed at normal running speeds.

In the last part of this lesson, I get clients to adjust their leg tension: to stiffen their legs to increase their cadence, and to soften their legs to reduce their cadence. They should find what's comfortable: where they bounce with the least effort. Once everyone is comfortably bouncing, they can look at each other and see that the whole-foot landing makes them vertically aligned too.

The technique of stiffening the legs upon landing will be a useful tool in refining their technique later in their transition.

Lesson Two—Take-off

The take-off lesson (Chapter 6) helps clients to start thinking and feeling that good technique is all about getting off the ground as easily as possible, and allowing their momentum to carry them forwards.

The most important part of the take-off lesson is using the bounce exercise (EXERCISE 6.1). Getting them used to 'bouncing and tilting' instead of 'walking' is the important point here. Remember to start clients off with a sideways tilt, as this helps to prevent them bending over at the waist. Then move them on to alternating between tilting backwards and forwards.

Once clients move on to using alternate feet, their legs need to be comfortably flexed: enough to bounce them efficiently with no obvious foot-lifting. This is important for the next exercise, where they start moving and are in danger of resuming old 'walking' habits.

The next important thing is moving off with good form. I begin by getting clients to bounce on both feet, and then alternate feet, while trying to keep the same bouncing action (EXERCISE 6.2). Once they start to move, they need to focus on the bouncing and gentle tilting, and this is why I include a series of 'backwards, forwards, backwards' tilts before I finally ask them to tilt very gently forwards to start running (EXERCISE 6.3). They need to know they are trying to get the hips away from the ground, not the feet, which will follow naturally.

Lesson Three—Accelerating

During the acceleration lesson (Chapter 7), it is important to explain to clients that all they need to do is put a little more energy into the take-off. Point out that good runners combine an extra upwards motion with their existing forwards movement instinctively.

A lot of clients bend forwards at the waist when they accelerate. I usually 'trick' clients into accelerating by telling them to 'take off a bit higher' soon after we have set off. It comes as a big surprise to them how much they accelerate when they try to go up!

Lesson Four—Keith's Game Changer

Keith's Game Changer (Chapter 8) is very successful and often produces a near-perfect running action almost immediately. The biggest problem clients can have is that they tilt forwards too much and tilt back again too quickly in the exercises (EXERCISE 8.1 and EXERCISE 8.2), so they go past their balance point and start over-striding. If they gradually reduce the 'kick' so that they ease towards vertical, they cannot miss the 'sweet spot' where they are perfectly balanced. Remember that after 4 to 6 attempts the tilting will have become very subtle.

Lesson Five—Going for a run

In this lesson (Chapter 9), I try to give readers of this book the support I would personally give to clients during my sessions by providing them with a set plan to follow when going for a run and several exercises to monitor their technique. At the same time, the exercises in this lesson can be used by coaches as the core of their sessions. Finally, at the end of this lesson, I have included the techniques to employ when running hills.

After going through Keith's Game Changer, continue with the warm-up exercises to check form: Starting Off (EXERCISE 9.1), the Back-foot Check (EXERCISE 9.2) and The 360-degree Spin (EXERCISE 9.3). Use these exercises to ensure clients start their run in a correct way. The Back-foot Check works well for most runners, especially heel-strikers, and The 360-degree Spin works for everyone, every time. After just one run-through, clients are usually ready to start finding the balance point while running, using the exercises in the next lesson.

Note: Teach clients how to run hills in the second or third session, after they are comfortable with running on the flat. In the chapters, I have included this at the end of Chapter 9 to complete the picture of a typical run where they encounter hills.

Lesson Six—Maintaining good form

The maintaining good form lesson (Chapter 10) contains a series of exercises that can be used to check and correct running form by getting clients to focus on different movements in a variety of situations.

The exercises in Section 10.1, *Ways to check your form during your run*, you can use with your clients on their first session. Those in Section 10.2, *Other checks and exercises to refine your form*, are generally exercises that your clients can do on their own. However, I usually get clients to run barefoot on a hard surface to show them a way of feeling more precision in their running. You might also show them EXERCISE 6.4, Single-leg Start, to encourage the 'Spring don't swing' rule (OYF Rule#5), especially if they have previously had a big over-stride.

At this point in the session, I conclude my lessons and listen to feedback and field questions from the class.

Post-session guidance

Once the coaching session is over, the discussion is usually about where to buy suitable shoes and how much training should be done. It is imperative that all clients fully understand that even a small change in their technique, or a change to lighter shoes, will make a big difference to muscle use. Please make sure that clients follow the guidelines in Chapter 12, *Managing your transition*.

It is also extremely important that your clients attend at least one follow-up session, and to make sure they do not adopt other techniques, especially those that will cause injury. Examples are toe-running, knee-lifting, foot-lifting or buying unsuitable shoes such as zero-drop shoes that can be up to 20 millimetres thick.

Finally, it is important to keep in touch with your clients via email, etcetera, and refer them to our website (olderyetfaster.com) or the book.

A.4 Coaching tips for common problems

Below are some common technique problems, and the exercises I find most useful for correcting these problems.

Heel-strikers

Heel-striking is the most common problem you will encounter. Try these remedies:

- *Keith's Game Changer* (Chapter 8) has the most effective exercises to fix this problem (EXERCISE 8.1 and EXERCISE 8.2), since it starts with landing on the forefoot with a high cadence and feet moving high off the ground. All these actions are the opposite to what clients do when heel-striking.
- The Back-foot Check (EXERCISE 9.2) works remarkably well too, as clients cannot lean back while doing this exercise.
- The Acceleration Ladder (EXERCISE 10.3) is also useful. First try getting clients to accelerate with a more powerful take-off.
- Tilting to accelerate also works well since clients will have spent years leaning back when landing. In this case, they should be encouraged to stand up 'like a broomstick' and tilt from the ankle joint. This crude method is quite effective in reducing the backwards leaning.

Toe-runners

Toe-runners are usually runners who have attempted to stop heel-striking. They make the same leg action (a swing or lift) and simply change the angle of their foot. This can be a tricky problem to overcome, as the runner will have consciously practised this action many thousands of times. You will find these tips useful in helping these clients:

- Use EXERCISE 6.4 (Single-leg Start) whole-foot hopping to reduce the 'toe-jamming' action.
- Use the Back-foot Check (EXERCISE 9.2).
- Use The Pendulum (EXERCISE 10.1 and EXERCISE 10.2) to encourage whole-foot landings and to refine your clients' balance upon landing.
- Ask your clients to practice accelerating by increasing the power of the take-off rather than by tilting.
- Encourage your clients to dorsiflex the back foot. See the note about symmetry in Section A.6, *General tips* below.
- Warn clients of the dangers of not rectifying toe-running, particularly metatarsal stress fractures. This is where videos are important, as clients probably won't notice when there is too much pressure on their forefoot.
- Encourage your clients to practice barefoot running on smooth concrete so they will adapt quicker.

Knee-lifters or 'lift-and-place runners'

Knee-lifting or 'lift-and-place running' is frequently a problem with barefoot runners. I also see hints of this with track runners who practice lifting their knees, reaching forwards and clawing back along the ground.

This type of running is perhaps caused by clients' misconception that arises when they view fast runners and sprinters and mistakenly think they have to lift their knees. Lifting the feet (and therefore the knees) will waste energy and ensure the runner leans back to do it!

The bounce-and-tilt exercises in lessons one (Chapter 5) and two (Chapter 6) are obviously good for these clients, as these exercises require them to take off rather than to walk along the ground. Apart from this solution, use the same exercises as for heel-strikers. Sometimes just getting the runner to stop actively lifting their knees by telling them to 'push their knees forwards, parallel to the ground' helps.

The Back-foot Check (EXERCISE 9.2) is also very useful as runners are unable to lift their feet in front of them when doing this exercise.

Back-foot lifters

Runners who lift their feet behind them tend to be toe-jammers, and both these problems should be fixed with Keith's Lessons, since the focus is on lifting the whole body rather than part of it. However, some runners persist. Encouraging them to simply leave their foot on the ground slightly longer often works well for these runners—long enough to prevent the foot being lifted, but not so long that it gets dragged. The Back-foot Check (EXERCISE 9.2) also has a good success rate, as does the Back-foot Adjustment (EXERCISE 10.4).

Arm- and shoulder-swingers

For arm- and shoulder-swingers, no action is necessary because upper-body rotation largely disappears when the clients' over-stride is reduced. For awareness of their rotation get the clients to clasp their hands behind their back for a few strides. Then, while their hands are still clasped, get them to raise their shoulders, so they are standing more upright. The rotation should reduce.

A.5 Private sessions

My private sessions are slightly different from group coaching sessions as, in addition to the instructions and exercises, I also take a side-view video of my clients' running action. At the end of the private session, I take another video to show clients how they have improved (see OYF Rule #1). As well as showing clients the most obvious signs of over-striding—i.e. where the foot is landing well in front of the hips—these videos can help clients see lots of other symptoms, such as:

- a knee lift or the foot being pushed forwards before take-off
- arms coming across the body, or shoulder rotation
- a fully straightened leg upon landing
- a big drop in the height of the hips after landing
- a big bend at the waist—from sinking after landing and pushing off hard to take off.

A.6 General tips

One other observation I have made is that the movements of runners are symmetrical in every plane.

- If your clients are reaching forwards and pointing their toes, then their back foot will be pointed and stretched out behind them with their sole facing up. By simply getting them to dorsiflex their back foot, they will stop reaching forwards with their front foot, and this will reduce their over-stride. This is demonstrated particularly well by looking at footprints on firm sand.
- If your clients' shoulders are rotating, then you know their lower body is also rotating; they are over-striding.
- If your clients bend over at the waist, then, to balance, they are swinging their legs forwards underneath them. If their whole body is tilted forwards, then they will be kicking their feet up behind them to balance.

Two fine adjustment tricks for later in clients' progress are:

- Slightly reducing their cadence occasionally during training to help them get used to a stronger take-off and more air time. This will be just one or two steps per minute, nothing drastic.
- Increasing their leg stiffness on landing. This produces a more vertical landing and a better elastic take-off.

A.7 Summary

If you use the lessons in this book, you should be able to substantially reduce your clients' over-stride in one session. Of equal importance, you should leave them with methods for ongoing self-improvement. I hope that my experiences described in this chapter make that process even easier, as I would like nothing better than for my technique-change methods to be adopted by coaches as the basis for improving their clients' running.

I invite you to test the lessons, use them and adapt them as you see fit. All I ask is that you acknowledge Heidi's and my work, and that you direct people to our website or this book. I am sure you will have as much success as I have; but, if you encounter any problems, do not be shy in coming forwards: I am always available to receive feedback. Good luck—make some great runners!

APPENDIX B
FOR PODIATRISTS—TREATING RUNNERS

Heidi Jones (Dip. Pod., MA. Pod. A)

I have included this appendix to show podiatrists a better way to treat injuries, and specifically runners' injuries. In this appendix, I explain how I assess my patients and how I help them using Heidi's Strengthening Program and my rehabilitation exercises. Before I elaborate on these, let me briefly establish some context.

In Australia, a podiatrist diagnoses, treats and prevents injuries to the feet and lower limbs. I qualified as a podiatrist back in 1996, and the following year I started work at the podiatry clinic of St Vincent's Hospital in Sydney. As you might remember, this was the time when diabetes first emerged as a major problem worldwide. As a consequence, the clinic redirected their resources into treating patients with diabetic foot ulcers. Three years later, I set up my own podiatry practice, 'Feet on the Move', which gave me experience with a wider variety of patients, a lot of whom presented with running injuries.

My professional training and my love of anatomy gave me a solid platform from which to develop Heidi's Strengthening Program, but two major factors drove me to actually create it. The first factor was that when the podiatrists treating my running injuries in the 1990s followed the 'accepted wisdom', especially with regard to orthotics, my injuries would—instead of getting better—increase. This forced me to look very closely at what was being taught in podiatry. Secondly, I had to fall back on my own resources to overcome this series of injuries. This led me to realise that it was strengthening the feet that allowed me and my patients to recover naturally and that, in most cases, orthotics were not needed.

Heidi's Strengthening Program grew from gathering the best remedies from a number of areas through my own experiences—such as the Spiky Ball exercise (EXERCISE 11.1) from self-myofascial release theory, and ballet exercises from my Pilates instructor. I then added some of the foot exercises from a running coach. I give full acknowledgements in Appendix C. Finally, Keith showed me how to run properly, and I was then able to understand good running biomechanics and apply it to my patients. Fortuitously, Heidi's Strengthening Program is also 'just what is needed' to help runners to transition when they change their running technique via Keith's Lessons.

B.1 The 'accepted wisdom'

We podiatrists are as time-poor as most other medical professionals: we deal with a steady stream of patients while trying to keep up to date with advances in medical knowledge and a myriad of other work-related tasks. We learn to cope, but sometimes we do not take enough time to look into the causes of our patients' problems, and we merely end up treating their symptoms (see OYF Rule#6). However, by doing this we are effectively saying that they have a permanent disability. Failing to identify and address the cause of their injury is setting them up for long-term treatment expenses and exposing them to further injury. Return visits are not in our best interests, nor in our patients'.

It does not help when information that we have been taught to rely on is incorrect. When it comes to treating runners' injuries, we are trained to fix their problems in the first instance by prescribing shoes and orthotics. The current textbook approach is to cushion and support runners' feet rather than to look further into the cause of their injuries, which, in the large majority of cases, will be due to incorrect running technique. If our patients continue to run badly and think they can fix this by using shoes and prescribed orthotics, they will be sorely mistaken. Not only will they find that their running will not improve, they will experience more injuries.

The main reason that podiatrists and physiotherapists start off on the wrong track is due to the continued acceptance of the biomechanical theories of Dr Merton Root, DPM (Doctor of Podiatric Medicine in the USA). He pioneered 'foot orthosis' technology in the late 1950s, experimenting with the new materials of thermoplastics in fashioning his orthotics. In 1971, along with his colleagues, he came up with the criteria for judging if a foot has structural defects and thus can be deemed 'abnormal'. In 1977, they published a textbook, *Normal and abnormal functions of the foot*, which is still used today as an important reference by many professionals. This is in spite of the fact that Dr Root's theories were seriously questioned in the 1990s. Some of the eight biophysical criteria that Dr Root used to define 'normal' foot structure have subsequently been shown to be inaccurate by Dr Kevin Kirby DPM.

In 1992, renowned American Podiatric Surgeon, Dr Kevin Kirby DPM, decided that it would be more productive to take an engineering approach when treating foot problems, rather than trying to compensate for Root-defined 'foot deformities'. He put his efforts into designing a mechanical therapy to reduce or eliminate stresses on the foot. This approach was a step forwards and moved away from measurement and foot types to basing treatment on foot pathology.

In 1995, Professor Thomas McPoil and Physical Therapist Gary Hunt further discussed the problems found in Root-defined foot biomechanics. They proposed the 'tissue stress model', which looks at the internal tissue stress rather than measuring and categorising the foot.

These researchers were on the right track, but Keith and I go a step further in this book by looking at how the running action influences the stresses that are put on the foot, as well as how the foot and the body absorb these stresses.

B.2 Questioning the 'accepted wisdom'

Two situations that we, podiatrists, face in the course of our work are, firstly a lack of relevant information, and secondly a situation where the accepted practice has never been questioned.

No doubt you have experienced a situation where a patient presents to you and you are unable to find the real cause of their problem. At the time, you don't have all the data that you need to make a correct diagnosis. This was the case for my podiatrist when I went to him with my initial foot problem. His prescription of orthotics was perfectly reasonable and based on the information that he had available to him.

However, my problem turned out to be due to a rare medical condition and required surgery. In these circumstances, nothing could have been done differently. The second problem occurred when I was advised to continue to use orthotics after I had my foot operated on to fix Freiberg's disease. As soon as I was able to walk, I could have done my foot exercises, but the accepted wisdom was orthotics. According to the theory, which is still unfortunately current, I continued to use orthotics, which only introduced other injuries.

In my running, orthotics changed my technique, which in turn caused me to over-pronate. To make matters worse, I was prescribed more orthotics to fix this, and this resulted in 15 years of painful running. All these injuries did not need to have happened. After the operation, I should have simply discarded my orthotics and gone back to my old running routine using thin, flat, flexible shoes. My big mistake was that I believed what I was taught. This story shows that we should always question prescribed doctrine and test it scientifically.

Don't get me wrong, both Keith and I realise the benefit of orthotics in certain instances. We know that there are many situations where orthotics are needed—sometimes permanently, as in the case of true foot deformities, or for high-risk diabetics with neuropathic feet that are prone to ulcers. There are also many instances where orthotics help in the short term; for example, where the foot needs support after an accident or an operation where the body has undergone a sudden change and has to adjust rapidly to the stress. What we object to is that orthotics are widely prescribed to address a range of foot pathologies and over-pronation in running, yet these problems are easily fixed by technique change, strengthening and running in thin, flat, flexible shoes.

Questionable theories taught as fact

Keith and I have found all the assertions listed below to be fallacious, and we have developed our own training methods accordingly. We have many, many satisfied clients who will attest to the efficacy of our work. The bottom line is that when fixing running problems, orthotics should only be prescribed as a last resort. Podiatrists and physiotherapists are taught incorrectly about both the running action and appropriate shoes.

Incorrect 'facts' about running technique:
- The first point of contact with the ground should be the heel.
- There are different types of landings (foot strikes).
- You can accurately assess a runner's gait from behind.

Incorrect 'facts' about shoes and orthotics:
- A runner needs cushioned and supportive shoes to run well or to prevent injury.
- A runner needs to choose a type of shoe that controls their foot action.
- A runner needs a certain type of shoe for their foot shape or imprint on a pressure plate.
- Orthotics are the way to minimise excessive pronation.

B.3 What should be taught

In podiatry, I come across a number of areas where the teaching is outdated or simply not correct. As mentioned earlier, the textbook *Normal and abnormal functions of the foot* is still used today as an important reference by many professionals. However, the measurement criteria this textbook uses are based on inaccuracies, and more advanced theories are only slowly being adopted.

The over-prescription of orthotics is a major problem. Many podiatrists have a default position of proposing orthotics to help with foot problems without considering other options. Sure, orthotics can give pain relief and may be required in some cases, but I find that in many other cases they are not required. Let us just look at two of the conditions that a patient may present with: 'flat feet' and 'high arches'. We are referring to low or high medial arches. An orthotic used for these two conditions can give passive relief, but will end up weakening the muscles and tendons of the foot. If there are no arthritic changes in the midfoot, a better approach is to use the exercises in Heidi's Strengthening Program to get the patient to strengthen the small muscles of the foot, and then for the patient to also strengthen the glutes.

Instead of interfering with the body's natural ability to repair itself, the program strengthens the affected areas and gives the body the freedom to adjust itself. Specifically, the arches will strengthen, which gives the patient permanent pain relief without damaging other parts of the body.

I suggest that best practice for podiatrists should follow these general principles:
- Learn from experience and be prepared to question existing theories.
- The body responds extremely well when you strengthen it.
- Don't be afraid to strengthen the foot rather than try to support it with orthotics.
- Almost all running injuries are technique and shoe related.
- The spine needs to be vertical to engage the postural muscles of the pelvis and torso (OYF Rule #2). The shoes must provide a stable base for this.
- As a podiatrist, you need to view patients from the side, rather than the back, to pick up any over-stride (OYF Rule #1).

B.4 Treating runners better

I start assessing my patients the moment they walk into the treatment room. Especially if they are runners, the three things I notice immediately are footwear, posture and muscular development. In that way, I can diagnose what they have been doing wrong in their running, and therefore how they have incurred their injury. This analysis combines what Keith taught me and my biomechanical knowledge. Of course, I also learn from my patients about their previous injuries, their running history, their current pain, and their future training plans. Although my patients always need to strengthen their muscles, this initial assessment gives me all the information I need to decide how much rehabilitation they need.

How I assess running injuries

When a runner comes to me for treatment, I usually know how to go about fixing their running injuries by the time they have finished describing them to me. I look at their body shape, the way they walk, their stance and the shoes they have on. The two main causes of injuries will be their running technique and the type of shoes they wear. It is amazing how much shoes influence runners' body shape.

Illustration 59, *figures A, B* and *C* shows how poor posture, induced by wearing shoes with a raised heel, changes the patient's proprioception, the sense of the relative position of their feet to the ground. A patient who has been walking on an angled surface for years, gets used to using the wrong muscle groups, and what the patient feels as upright is not.

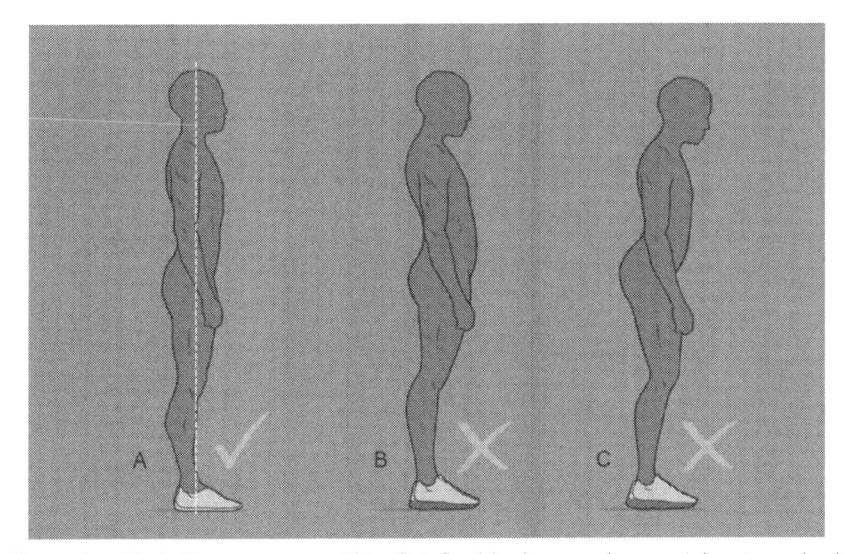

Illustration 59: A. Correct posture. Thin, flat, flexible shoes and an upright, strong body with postural muscles engaged. B. Incorrect posture. Raising the heel makes you push your knees back and your hips forwards. C. Incorrect posture. Raising the heel makes you bend your knees and your lower back. In neither B nor C the spine is vertical.

This use of the wrong muscle group and incorrect body alignment leads to short-term and long-term changes to the body. This is why the patient's footwear forms a vital part of my assessment process. Therefore, I ask patients to bring with them the shoes they wear casually, for work and for running. This enables me to teach them that, simply by buying suitable footwear and following Heidi's Strengthening Program, they can recover and not re-injure themselves.

Whether a runner or not, wearing unsuitable shoes is extremely damaging to the body. The short-term damaging effects to the feet when wearing a shoe with a raised heel and a turned-up toe box manifest in ailments, such as plantar fasciitis, metatarsalgia, and shortening of the Achilles tendon. With the foot held in this artificial position, the body weight is shifted forwards onto the metatarsal heads. In the long term, bony changes occur as the metatarsal heads drop, because the metatarsophalangeal joint (the joint at the base of the toe and the metatarsal head) is in a fixed plantarflexed position. This partial dislocation results in clawed-toe deformities and arthritic changes to the forefoot. Wearing shoes with a raised heel will also exacerbate hallux adbucto valgus deformity. The intrinsic muscles of the foot become weakened because they cannot function in this position, and this causes malalignment further up the body.

As shown in *Illustration 59*, when wearing a shoe with a raised heel, the spine is no longer vertical. This creates long-term problems because the postural muscles of the trunk (abdominals, erector spinate and gluteus medius) cannot engage in this position. These muscles then become weak due to lack of use, and this leads to stress in areas such as the lower back and the neck. In runners, the changed posture, together with the influence of the shoes leads to a high-impact running technique, and hence to the running injuries that we all see on a daily basis.

I complete my assessment and diagnosis by the usual method of asking my patients detailed questions about where they have pain and applying my knowledge of anatomy and podiatry. I then go one step further by drawing on my own experience with running injuries and my understanding of running technique. I determine how much strengthening and rehabilitation they need for their treatment and I make sure they have suitable footwear, before explaining to them how to sort out their running action. My holistic approach not only fixes their problems, but also improves their running technique, which helps to prevent them incurring future injuries. They tell me 'It makes so much sense!'

Heidi's Strengthening Program

Heidi's Strengthening Program, which is my standard treatment for fixing foot problems, is set out in Chapter 11, and explained in more detail in Appendix C.

I start with strengthening the feet using the Spiky Ball and Foot Program exercises (see Section 11.1, *Strengthening your feet*) to massage, stretch and strengthen patients' feet and ankles, and to some extent their calf muscles. My Quarter Knee Squat (EXERCISE 11.8) is then used to strengthen their gluteus medius.

Heidi's Strengthening Program is meant to help patients recover from injuries as well as strengthen their feet, calves and glutes. The exercises also provide the strengthening that is essential to prevent injuries when clients are changing their running technique via Keith's Lessons.

My Spiky Ball and Foot Program exercises, when combined with a change to thin, flat, flexible footwear have excellent results. The patient normally needs only one visit and I am amazed at how quickly their feet are strengthened. The program is so good that I now give it to non-runners, and always to children. I start by taking my patients through the exercises specific for their situation and I follow up by emailing them videos of their exercises, so that they are more likely to do them. I encourage them to keep in touch with me, so I can follow up and monitor their progress. I also provide them with suggestions for appropriate footwear, which will not only be suitable for running, but also for work, school and casual wear. Unfortunately, it is often necessary to write to schools, so children are allowed to wear non-supportive, flat shoes.

The Spiky Ball and Foot Program exercises rehabilitate many injuries, including:

- Achilles tendonitis
- Achilles tendinosis
- plantar fasciitis
- calf muscle pain
- Morton's neuroma
- metatarsalgia
- anterior shin splints
- peroneal tendonitis
- medial tibial stress syndrome
- ankle pain
- subluxed cuboid
- posterior tibial tendonitis
- paediatric flat foot
- miserable malalignment syndrome
- Sever's disease
- stress fractures of the foot and lower leg.

My Quarter Knee Squat (EXERCISE 11.8) not only provides an excellent way of assessing patients, but also rehabilitates patients and is essential in strengthening their gluteus medius and core muscles. The first thing to assess is the patient's gluteus medius strength, since this is an area where runners need to be strong. Many of them come to me being surprisingly weak and this is immediately evident when I get them to take off their shoes and do this exercise with their torso vertical. It is remarkable how most fail this test, even though you would expect them to be using the necessary muscles all the time. Patients typically bend forwards at the waist, their hip drops on the non-weight-bearing side, and their knee collapses inward. They rarely can do ten squats, let alone 30, at the first go. If they cannot stand stable on one leg, doing this simple test, how can they expect to train without injury? Some are even entered in marathons!

This running-specific exercise is an essential rehabilitation exercise for Achilles tendonitis and tendinosis, posterior tibial tendonitis and knee injuries, but can only be used when the patient is able to weight bear on the injured leg without pain.

The exercise will strengthen the gluteus medius, iliopsoas and vastus medius obliquus, which need to work in unison during the weight-bearing phase of running. Patients who are in this situation are my favourite cases to work on, because they adapt so quickly to strengthening and technique change. Although they almost always fail at first, they respond very well to this one exercise after some practice. To see how the Quarter Knee Squat should be done, see Chapter 11, *Illustration 44* and the videos at olderyetfaster.com.

For a runner, it is essential that their glutes are strong, as weak glutes will result in a number of problems throughout the body such as:

- excessive hip-drop
- internal rotation of the femur causing maltracking of the patella
- excessive pronation, which in turn stresses the Achilles tendon, the posterior tibialis tendon, and all the stabilising muscles of the lower leg.

When runners are told that they have weak glutes, a physiotherapist will often put them through a vigorous strengthening program. Unfortunately, if they are running badly, they will resume their over-striding and, as these strengthened muscles will quickly atrophy, the gain in strength will be lost. This is extremely frustrating for the patient after so much hard work, especially when their injuries come back.

The Quarter Knee Squat is vital in rehabilitation, as it strengthens the gluteus medius and helps with the following problems:

- knee pain (VMO strengthening)
- hip pain
- Achilles tendonitis
- posterior tibial tendonitis
- other injuries that have resulted from weak glutes
- back pain from poor footwear (accidental bonus)
- neck pain from poor footwear (accidental bonus).

Case study 1

FUNCTIONAL ORTHOTICS PRESCRIBED FOR FLAT FEET

I came across a 40-year-old runner who had been prescribed functional orthotics for over 30 years, ever since he was a young school boy, due to flat feet. He even wore orthotics in his slippers. After reading our book, he sought out Keith for a technique session. Understandably, his feet and calf muscles were extremely sore, and he came to me for help too.

Patient history

A detailed history revealed that his training and racing had always been sabotaged by one over-striding injury after another. For example, chondromalacia patellae (runner's knee), iliotibial band friction syndrome, bursitis of the hip, and hip flexor pain.

Examination

He brought his supportive running shoes and several pairs of orthotics that his previous podiatrist had prescribed. I asked him to put them on and took a photo of him from the side. I then took a photo of him without shoes, also from the side.

When he had his supportive shoes and orthotics on, his hips were shifted forwards, his knees were pushed back and he had an excessive lordotic curve. When in bare feet, his hips were still shifted forwards and his spine still had that lordotic curve. He was so weak that he could not stand straight. His feet were hypermobile and so flat that there was no discernible arch and he had calcaneal eversion on stance, with classic soft-tissue bulge. There were no arthritic changes in the midfoot.

Treatment

I explained to this patient that it would take him more than two years for his body to fully strengthen and asked him, was this something he wanted to do? He was extremely keen and I took him on board.

I took him through Heidi's Strengthening Program (Chapter 11) and got him into thin, flat, flexible shoes for all activities—something he has passed on to his young family. We kept in contact and, months later, I invited him to join our informal Sunday Run Group, which is for our book readers who want to further improve their technique.

Patient's recovery

It took approximately eight months before his calf muscle soreness started to subside. It was then that he started experiencing posterior tibial tendon soreness, which lingered for six months. Fifteen months into his transition, his arches in his feet started to develop and he had associated tightness in his peroneal muscles. They were being stretched for the first time!

Now, two years later, he is standing vertically aligned and cannot tolerate shoes with even a 2 or 3 millimetre drop. Keith and I have also noticed a dramatic improvement in his running technique, and we see associated development of his abdominal and gluteal muscles.

Without any speed work and only three runs per week, totalling 15 kilometres, he ran a 5-kilometre local park run in 18 minutes 26 seconds. This shows how important good running technique is. I am honoured to be part of this patient's journey and excited to watch him reach his potential as an athlete.

What I have learnt from treating this condition

Whether the patient is a child or an adult, the current treatment for flat feet is functional orthotics. However, there needs to be a distinction between a true flat foot deformity and a functioning flat foot. I have shown in this instance, and many others, that the foot responds very well to strengthening, and that this provides the patient with a permanent solution and an improved quality of life.

Case study 2

> ### A COMPLICATED CASE OF PLANTAR FASCIITIS, BILATERAL MEDIAL MENISCUS PAIN AND LOWER BACK PAIN
>
> #### Patient history
>
> This patient was a part-time farmer who was extremely frustrated, as he had tried several pairs of orthotics over years of treatment for plantar fasciitis without success.
>
> #### Examination
>
> Not only did this patient still have plantar fasciitis, but he also suffered from medial meniscus pain in both knees (if the orthotics over-supinate the feet, they impinge the medial aspect of the knee), and his lower back hurt. The shoes he presented in, and the boots he wore on the farm, had raised heels and turned-up toe boxes. This footwear design loaded the plantar fascia and put his whole skeleton out of alignment.
>
> #### Treatment
>
> When a patient presents to me with multiple injuries, I always start off with their feet and work up.
>
> Firstly, I advised him to immediately discard his orthotics. Not only were they weakening his feet, but they over-supinated both subtalar joints, stressing the medial meniscus in both of his knees. By pronating the subtalar joints, medial meniscus relief is immediate.
>
> I then showed him how to roll out his feet with the spiky ball and this took the pain away from his plantar fascia. I followed this exercise with my Foot Program, and his pleasure was now evident in his sparkling bright eyes! I got him to wear thin, flat, flexible shoes for both during the day and when he was on the farm. The flat shoes take the pressure off the plantar fascia and allow the toes to be flat on the ground. This engages the intrinsic muscles of the feet, which is important for balance. Further up the skeleton, wearing flat shoes reduces the pressure at the knee joint and the lower back, and enables the spine to be vertical. In

this position, the postural muscles of the trunk are able to fully engage, which keeps the upper body strong.

The next step—after he did my Spiky Ball and Foot Program exercises (see Section 11.1, *Strengthening your feet*) daily for a month—was to strengthen his vastus medius obliquus (VMO), the main knee-stabilising muscle (see EXERCISE 13.3). The leg extensions needed to be slow and controlled. He did three sets of 20, twice daily. His program started with a 2 kilogram weight and worked up to 3 kilogram over the month. Some patients might have to work through a little pain for this exercise (this is the only exercise where this is the case).

Once completely free from knee pain, the final step was to strengthen his gluteus medius with my Quarter Knee Squat. He did three sets of ten exercises, once per day for six weeks.

Patient's recovery

His plantar fascia healed in 6 weeks. It took 6 months for his knee pain to subside. It took another 6 weeks of gluteus medius strengthening for his lower back pain to disappear. He contacted me a year later to say he is still pain free.

What I have learnt from treating this condition

The combination of flat shoes and VMO strengthening has remarkable results for knee pain. Remember, however, that knee injuries can sometimes take many months to fully heal; though the great thing is that this treatment is not a temporary fix.

Once your patient can stand on one leg without pain, the final step is to strengthen their gluteus medius muscle. This is vital for pelvic stability during both walking and running. For non-runners, I prescribe three sets of 10 quarter knee squats on each leg and, for runners, I build up to three sets of 30.

When a patient presents with joint pain—whether knee or lower back—the first thing I do is to get them to wear thin, flat, flexible shoes and do the strengthening exercises. This won't work for everyone, but it is the easiest method to start off with. I am continually surprised at how effective it is.

Case study 3

LEARNING FROM MY OWN INJURIES

If you have read my story, you will know I am a lifelong runner who encountered some serious injuries.

I started experiencing early symptoms of Freiberg's disease in 1990 and a word-of-mouth referral led me to the late great podiatrist Philip Vasyli. I hobbled into his office, unable to weight bear on my second metatarsophalangeal joint. While sitting in his examination chair, he pushed firmly, on the sole of my foot, proximal to my second metatarsal head. As he did that, he extended my second toe and it moved easily with no pain. He then made me a thin orthotic, carefully placing a metatarsal dome to take the pressure off the affected area. He put me on a treadmill and it was pure bliss, I could run with no pain. Phil was very impressed with my running technique and he said I was the 'straightest runner he had ever seen'. I thought this man was a god and my career choice was now decided. I was hooked. I wanted to be a podiatrist and fix other runners like Phil did.

I was pain free for 12 months before the Freiberg's infarction fully manifested. Nothing Phil could do would fix this and I was in deep trouble. In 1992, the correct diagnosis of Freiberg's disease was made and successfully operated on by Dr Kim Slater. By now, Phil had moved overseas and his successor advised me to continue wearing orthotics. By 1995, I was able to resume running and I followed this advice; but, unknown to me, the orthotics were forcing me into an over-stride. By this time, running shoes had become chunkier and more supportive than my old flat shoes. To top it off, I was studying podiatry and we were taught in biomechanics class that the first point of contact was the heel. Wanting to be a good runner again, I perfected this biomechanically unsound and damaging technique. I was no longer the 'straightest runner' Philip Vasyli had ever seen.

My injuries and treatment

I was constantly told that I over-pronated and was therefore prescribed progressively more rigid and higher orthotics as a cure.

This created a downward spiral and eventually my body broke down!

Six months into training, I sustained the first of a series of tibial stress fractures. Eventually, after the seventh fracture, I discarded the orthotics, at which point the stress fractures stopped. I had persisted with orthotics for 15 painful years, all the time believing in what I was taught in college. However, I still wore supportive running shoes—which is still the current teaching—and I continued to suffer, with a further seven years of over-striding injuries.

I was constantly stiff in my shoulders and my neck, and I went through all the classic over-striding injuries—chondromalacia patellae (runner's knee), iliotibial band friction syndrome, hip flexor pain, bursitis of the hip. I also had weak stomach muscles and a lordotic/kyphotic curve, all of which was put down to me being hypermobile. I now realise my skeleton was out of alignment and I had a weak core due to years of wearing shoes with a raised heel. It took six months of daily Pilates sessions to be able to engage my deep abdominal muscles.

My recovery

I moved back into flatter shoes after meeting Keith, and he changed my technique back to what it was when I was a teenager. Things began to improve, but it took two years of wearing flat shoes before my chronic back and neck pain fully subsided. Now, my spine is straight and my calf, gluteus medius and other postural muscles are all strong. I haven't suffered any over-striding injuries since and I feel great after every run.

Interesting clinical points

When I first presented to Philip Vasyli, my arches were well developed, possibly from running barefoot at my local Little Athletics club. I distinctly remember Phil saying I had a 'forefoot valgus'. It was such an odd term to me that it stayed in my head.

After wearing orthotics and supportive shoes with a raised heel for five years, I was reassessed in my biomechanical class at podiatry college. I had a forefoot varus, calcaneal eversion and

> miserable malalignment syndrome with bilateral squinting patella and lordosis and kyphosis.
>
> Two years after wearing flat shoes and doing my strengthening program, my feet were again strong, my legs and back had straightened up, and I was pain free.
>
> What I have learnt from my experiences
>
> In certain circumstances, orthotics can be effective in the short term; but prolonged use will be detrimental to posture and running technique, and therefore cause secondary injuries. It was a frustrating, expensive, depressing waste of time for me, which could have been avoided if I had simply fixed my running action, run in the proper shoes with no raised heel or orthotics, and strengthened my feet.
>
> I see patients every day who are heading in the same direction, or who are already suffering chronic pain, and it is my experiences that have given me the skill and confidence to treat these patients simply and effectively.

Plantar fasciitis and orthotics—a sad story

While running a workshop at Southampton Athletic Club (United Kingdom), I met a runner who had been prescribed orthotics for plantar fasciitis. Within a few weeks, he suffered from severe knee pain and, despite going back to his podiatrist several times, the podiatrist checked him from behind, said that 'he was straight', and was adamant he had to get used to them.

Two weeks later he tore the medial meniscus in both knees, required emergency surgery and was out from running for a year.

This sad example illustrates that when the podiatrist prescribes orthotics that over-supinate the subtalar joint, these impinge the medial aspect of the knee joint, stressing the medial meniscus. Also, as the orthotics raise the heel, the knee becomes stressed, especially when running. This forces the runner into an over-stride, which we now know is detrimental to the running action and extremely damaging to the body. Sadly, I see examples of this far too often.

What I have learnt from this runner

In the vast majority of cases such as this, all that is needed to convert to pain-free running is the correct shoes and good technique, combined with foot- and leg-strengthening exercises.

APPENDIX C
HEIDI'S STRENGTHENING PROGRAM EXPLAINED

Heidi Jones

As I was writing the chapter *Heidi's Strengthening Program*, I began to feel that there was a lot more to be said about the exercises, and about how Heidi's Strengthening Program evolved over the years. In this appendix, I describe the exercises in more depth for medical professionals and interested runners, and explain why the exercises should be done in a particular sequence. I also give full acknowledgement details of the people who have provided me with such great help along the way.

C.1 How I developed Heidi's Strengthening Program

I have already detailed my story in other sections (see *About the authors* and Appendix B), so just a quick recap here to give context as to why I was ideally placed to develop a program to help runners handle their injury problems.

I started my learning curve from an early age when I started to run in races. I had an operation to fix a genetic foot disease, and I then overcame a series of running injuries, which were only made worse by continuing to use orthotics. In the end, I discarded the orthotics and, with Keith's help, learnt to run well in proper shoes.

In 2006, I gathered together a series of exercises and started to use them to treat my patients. Over the years, I continued to improve and refine them and, in 2012, I added Alan McCloskey's foot exercises. In the following year, Keith started asking me about foot and leg structures in relation to his own biomechanics, and I began writing out treatment exercise programs for my patients so they could refer to them at home. Therefore, when the need for input into Keith's book came, I was ready to formalise these exercises. The process had taken me seven years, but in the end it resulted in Heidi's Strengthening Program, of which I am justly proud. I know it works and I have enjoyed seeing many patients relieved of injury and pain in the long term. In April 2013, Keith's Lessons and Heidi's Strengthening Program came together and culminated in OYF Running, and my co-authoring the first edition of this book *Older Yet Faster*.

C.2 Acknowledgements to my sources

I would like to more fully acknowledge the dedicated professionals and friends who influenced me the most. These people are gurus in their fields and I have the utmost respect for, and deep gratitude towards, them for their generosity and friendship.

Angelo Castiglione

(Spiky Ball exercise)

Angelo has 20 years' experience as an exercise professional and strength and conditioning coach. He is the founder of 180 Degrees Wellness (180degrees.com.au) and teaches the self-myofascial release therapy. I first met Angelo when I attended a one-day workshop he was presenting. Right from the start, I loved the spiky ball and I could see how useful it would be. It does so much for the foot and is the logical starting point for foot exercises. I always start my program with it.

Gaetano del Monaco

(Foot exercises from ballet: The Maestro, Birdie on a Wire, and Foot Bridges)

Gaetano was my Pilates teacher, but he is also an ex-professional ballet dancer, which is where he learnt the three exercises he showed me. I was referred to Gaetano by my exasperated massage therapist as, despite weekly massages, I suffered from chronic pain in my back, shoulders and neck and had constantly tight hip flexors. Gaetano guided me towards starting a foot program for my patients.

Alan McCloskey

(Toe Wave and Marble Mover foot exercises)

Alan is a running coach and a barefoot runner who coaches people who want to try barefoot running. He thinks, as we do, that if runners get the technique right they will stay injury free and run better. I met Alan in April 2013 at a running forum in Newcastle, New South Wales, where Keith was one of the panel of experts. We talked about feet from my perspective and from his, and he kindly showed me his favourite two foot exercises, which I use to complete my Foot Program.

Dr Christopher Jones

(Straight Leg – Bent Leg Calf Raise rehabilitation exercise)

Dr Chris Jones has been practising as an osteopath since 2002 (chrisjonesosteo.com.au). He has not only worked with elite athletes at the Australian Institute of Sport, but has also been an elite 800-metre runner himself. He is well respected, has presented at international conferences and published papers in medical journals.

C.3 Heidi's Strengthening Program under the microscope

I have put a lot of thought into creating a reliable system of exercises, which have proven to work in curing many injuries and in helping runners to transition to good technique.

There are three stages to Heidi's Strengthening Program:
- rolling out the plantar fascia
- strengthening the foot
- strengthening the glutes.

Rolling out the plantar fascia

Whether you are doing my program to strengthen or to repair your feet, the first thing you need to do is to loosen up your plantar fascia.

The Spiky Ball

The Spiky Ball (EXERCISE 11.1) is a massage that requires a hard spiky ball, about 10 centimetres in diameter, and involves placing your foot on top of the ball and rolling the sole of your foot over it.

The Spiky Ball exercise will benefit people suffering pain associated with plantar fasciitis, dealing with Achilles tendonitis and tendinosis injuries, and also anyone with tight muscles, looking to improve their flexibility, and circulation.

The reason why this exercise is so beneficial is that it simultaneously releases the plantar fascia, the myofascia, as well as every muscle, tendon and ligament attachment on the sole of the foot.

The plantar fascia is the thick portion of web-like tissue—called an aponeurosis—that runs down the middle of the foot in three bands (see *Illustration 60*).

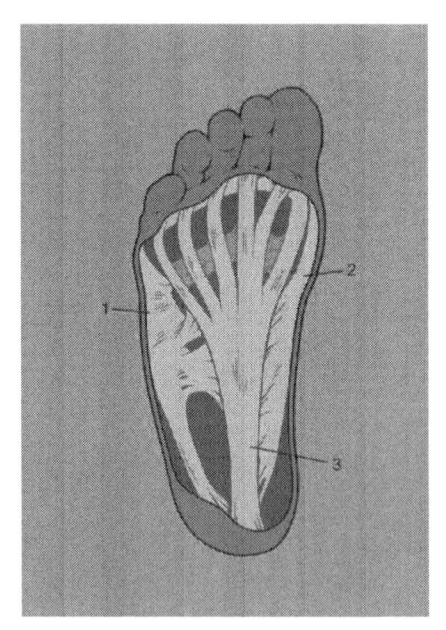

Illustration 60: Parts of the plantar fascia (aponeurosis). 1. Lateral band, 2. Medial band, 3. Central band.

From the heel, the plantar fascia branches out to the toes and supports the longitudinal arch of the foot. It is a resilient structure that supports and assists movement in the body. Like tendons, aponeuroses are made of collagen, but instead of a narrow band, they are shaped like a strong flat 'sheet' with a wide area of attachment that anchors them to the part that is moved by the attached muscle. However, while tendons allow the body to move and be flexible, aponeuroses allow the body to be strong and stable. They act like a spring that bears pressure and tension. Releasing the plantar fascia is therefore beneficial and provides relief for sufferers of most foot injuries.

The myofascia is the exceptionally strong, dense, flexible tissue that surrounds all muscles and bones. By releasing the myofascia, the Spiky Ball exercise relieves muscle soreness and joint stress, breaks up knots in muscles, and improves neuro-muscular efficiency (brain-to-foot communication).

A massage with the spiky ball also improves joint range-of-motion in the foot and ankle and, because part of the myofascia connects the underside of the foot with the ankle and calf muscle, can also relieve tight calf muscles, stiff ankles and Achilles tendon injuries. It simultaneously provides another benefit by engaging the gluteus medius muscle on the weight-bearing leg.

Strengthening the foot

After the plantar fascia has been rolled out and the foot is flexible and supple, I start my patients on my Foot Program exercises. First off is The Maestro, which works the foot-stabilising muscles. These are the supinators and pronators. We then work our way along different areas of the foot from non-weight-bearing to weight-bearing exercises, before ending with a standing stretch of the shin and ankle.

The first three exercises (The Maestro, Birdie on a Wire, and Foot Bridges) are done in a seated position (that is, non-weight-bearing), and all exercises involve both the feet and the lower leg—except the Foot Bridges exercise, which is isolated to the intrinsic muscles of the foot. As in ballet, all of the foot exercises intensely work the part of the foot that they apply to and involve using the whole foot.

The Maestro

The Maestro (EXERCISE 11.2) involves a large motion of the foot, firstly up and in, and then down and away. We are inverting and everting the feet to their end-of-range of motion and, at each end, we hold the pose and separate the toes for a greater stretch. This is extremely fatiguing.

The movement is in two planes and allows the greatest flexibility in the ankle joints. It stretches and strengthens the supinator and pronator muscles and tendons, and gives the full range-of-motion to the ankle joint. The movement gently works the Achilles tendon and stretches both sides of the plantar fascia. It also creates space between the metatarsal heads, which provides relief from Morton's neuroma.

Birdie on a Wire

By curling the toes and pointing the feet, Birdie on a Wire (EXERCISE 11.3) helps to realign dropped metatarsal heads. We are focusing on the forefoot and doing an intense workout of the front of the shin muscle. This exercise stretches out the Achilles tendon a bit more and involves the calf muscle. It also stretches and strengthens the extensor tendons on the top of the foot. I find that there is a strong correlation between patients wearing shoes with a raised heel and a turned-up toe box, and feet with dropped metatarsal heads.

Foot Bridges

In Foot Bridges (EXERCISE 11.4), we work the intrinsic muscles of the foot. These muscles are responsible for the integrity of the medial longitudinal, lateral longitudinal and transverse arches, and the balance and strength of the whole foot. This exercise requires a degree of concentration, so as not to engage the muscles of the legs at the same time. It is a finely controlled, small movement that requires brain-to-foot communication. When doing this exercise, patients may have to concentrate hard, but the benefit of doing this exercise is enormous. These muscles are only engaged when the toes touch the ground. Having the toes touching the ground is necessary for achieving good balance, which is why correct footwear is so important.

Toe Wave

We then move on to a weight-bearing exercise. The Toe Wave (EXERCISE 11.5) involves an intense workout of the tibialis anterior and a gentle stretch of the calf muscle and the Achilles tendon. This exercise also strengthens the forefoot, which will, in future, help with doing the Foot Bridges exercise.

Marble Mover

The Marble Mover (EXERCISE 11.6) is an intense workout that strengthens the three peroneal muscles (the pronators), as well as the posterior tibialis muscle and tendon, which is the main supinator of the foot. Strength here is vital for a good rebound during running. Although the posterior tibialis has been used in other exercises, it is only here that patients will feel it working. This exercise is particularly good for people who have been wearing supportive shoes or orthotics, as it will strengthen their weakened arches. This exercise also strengthens the ankle and the Achilles tendon.

Front of Shin and Ankle Stretch

The Front of Shin and Ankle Stretch (EXERCISE 11.7) is an exercise that specifically focuses on the front of the shin and the front of the ankle joint. The exercise engages the anterior tibialis muscle, and the extensor tendons on the top of the foot. It stretches the front of the ankle, giving full range-of-motion and flexibility to the joint. The exercise is a must for Achilles tendonitis and plantar fasciitis, as the tight fascia associated with these injuries causes the ankle joint to become 'stuck'.

Exercising the glutes

The gluteus medius, along with the gluteus maximus and the gluteus minimus, is one of a group of three muscles in the buttocks that are known collectively as the gluteal muscles, or simply referred to as the 'glutes'. These muscles originate from the ilium and sacrum, and attach to the femur. The gluteus medius provides stability and levels the hips, stopping the hips from dropping at one side and internally rotating.

Note that, if patients have weak glutes, they will most likely need to do my Spiky Ball and Foot Program exercises and my Quarter Knee Squat daily for six weeks before recommencing running.

Quarter Knee Squat

My Quarter Knee Squat (EXERCISE 11.8) is a very effective exercise that I developed to fix my own running problems. When I was running with orthotics, I realised that I had excessive hip-drop. To counteract this, I experimented with some exercises and came up with my Quarter Knee

Squat. It strengthened my glutes and has also worked extremely well for my patients over the years.

This exercise mimics the weight-bearing phase of running when the foot is on the ground and 'fully loaded'. As the foot lands, the hips lower to about one quarter of the length of the shin bone before rebounding off the ground. In this exercise, I slow this action right down and build balance and strength in the gluteus medius, iliopsoas, and the vastus medius obliquus as they work in unison.

About 80% of runners who come to see me have trouble doing this exercise. If they can't do this exercise without wobbling, the likelihood of sustaining an injury is very high.

APPENDIX D
SUMMARY OF OYF RULES

Keith Bateman and Heidi Jones

The OYF Rules emphasise the important aspects of what we are teaching.

OYF Rule #1: Get a side-view video regularly

You might think your foot is already landing under your hips, but you will find that in most instances it certainly is not. The only way to identify the extent of your over-stride is to take a side-view video. A front or back-view video will not show the over-stride and are largely irrelevant.

Ask a friend to take a video of you running at constant speed. Once you have the video, choose a frame where your foot has full pressure against the ground. Draw a vertical line through the centre of that ground-contact point. If your hips are behind the line, then you are leaning back and braking. Compare your results with *Illustration 18*, which shows perfectly aligned landing and the aligned take-off position that will produce it.

Continue to take side-view videos regularly throughout your transition.

OYF Rule #2: Stand and land aligned

The aim is for your spine to be vertical, which means you will engage the postural muscles of your stomach (abdominals), back (erector spinae) and bottom (gluteals). You should be in this upright stance whenever you are standing, walking or running and it can only be achieved by wearing thin, flat, flexible shoes. When running, you can only land aligned if you have such shoes.

By following this rule, you will build up all your muscles in the right proportions—calves, glutes, back, stomach, neck—every muscle you use will build as required. If you have spent decades in shoes that are raised up at the heel, then your muscles will have developed (and under-developed) to accommodate your non-vertical stance, and it will take some time for your body to re-adjust.

OYF Rule #3: Over-pronation is a symptom of over-striding

Your foot pronates throughout the whole landing. When you over-stride, landing takes much longer than normal and this causes over-pronation.

Blocking pronation (the foot rolling inward on landing) with supportive shoes or orthotics will force you to continue to damage your body with high-impact landings, and put undue stress across your whole body.

By following Keith's Lessons in this book, you will reduce any over-pronation you have by decreasing your over-stride. Being upright (OYF Rule #2) will strengthen your feet and your glutes and make sure over-pronation is never a problem again.

OYF Rule #4: Bounce and fly

Once you have mastered good running technique, you will naturally run faster and you will be surprised that your training times improve with no extra effort.

By simply concentrating on a balanced landing, you will continually reduce your braking and at the same time make yourself strong in the right places. This will make you land well and close to vertically aligned, with all your postural muscles naturally engaged. Then, once landed, the elasticity in your feet and legs will bounce you to a long stride and make you run faster.

OYF Rule #5: Spring, don't swing

By 'spring, don't swing' we mean do not swing your legs, or try to lift your knees or feet.

The 'spring' part comes from the elastic energy in an unrestricted foot and Achilles tendon, and is the result of landing balanced. The spring produces an immediate take-off in a slightly more forwards direction. In efficient running, getting airborne is natural and seems effortless (OYF Rule #4).

The more you need to push off when at constant speed, the more you will have braked upon landing. However, the best runners have very little 'drive': they quickly 'bounce' their body off their whole foot after landing near-vertically aligned with minimal braking.

OYF Rule #6: Fix the problem not the symptom

There is only one thing you need to fix in running: your over-stride.

Simply by reducing this, you will learn to land more balanced and you will start to fix everything else. This is because almost all injuries, and lack of speed, are due to your foot landing too far in front of you.

Trying to fix the symptom of over-striding with artificial supports, orthotics, 'special' shoes and so on, will just obscure the problem, allowing you to run badly for longer. You will continue to suffer.

OYF Rule #7: Hips first—your foot will follow

The majority of runners lift or swing their legs forwards, which causes their hips to be behind their foot when they land. The way of overcoming this problem is to 're-program' your brain to focus on your back foot catching up with your hips, rather than advancing your front foot.

The position you are looking for once you have fully landed is the position in the middle: neither leaning forwards or back. Don't make the mistake of pushing your hips forwards—just leave your foot on the ground and let your hips freely move ahead.

Using a side-view video (OYF Rule #1), compare your results with *Illustration 18*, which shows perfectly aligned landing and the aligned take-off position that will produce it. To keep a check on your progress and to make sure you are running with good form, continue to take a side-view video regularly.

OYF Rule #8: Don't try to control your feet

A good runner's feet will rise off the ground—but are not lifted—and land in a particular way—but not forced. Similarly, your feet should rise naturally and there should be an almost instant whole-foot landing that is observed and felt, but not controlled. This will happen when you land balanced.

Specifically:

- Don't try to place your feet on the ground.
- Don't lift your feet.
- Don't try to land on any part of your foot: inside, outside, toes or heel.
- Don't extend your stride length by reaching forwards with your feet.
- Don't try to reduce your over-stride by doing faster, shorter steps.

OYF Rule #9: Aim for balanced whole-foot landings

A whole-foot landing is an important step in getting a balanced landing, as it gives you good feedback on your technique. You should feel even pressure between your forefoot and your heel. Bring your awareness to this contact of your foot on the ground until you have managed to correct your technique.

At low speed, your heel will land firmly on the ground; you will feel a harsh, jarring sensation (think of a kangaroo hopping slowly). Once you speed up to about 6 minutes per kilometre, your landings will be much softer. You will eventually find the speed where it is even more efficient and you get a 'floating' feeling. For us, this starts at about 5 minutes per kilometre. Running starts to feel almost effortless as we approach 4 minutes per kilometre.

In every run you will be a little off-balance at times—even the best runners won't manage a perfect landing every time. You might feel the ball of your foot or your heel touch a little too firmly; but, on average, you should feel your whole foot giving you complete support. However, do not make the mistake of 'placing' your foot on the ground or you will over-stride.

OYF Rule #10: Drills and exercises should directly relate to the running action

If you are trying to strengthen or rehabilitate after injury, then the most useful drills and exercises are those that most closely resemble the running action—many do not. For instance, glute-strengthening exercises should be done on one leg, in a standing position. Otherwise you are not being specific enough for strengthening the muscles you need for running. Use drills where you can land whole-foot as much as possible and don't skid when you land.

APPENDIX E
KILOMETRES TO MILES CONVERSION CHART

MINUTES PER KILOMETRE	MINUTES PER MILE
3:00	4:48
3:08	5:00
3:15	5:12
3:17	5:15
3:26	5:30
3:30	5:36
3:35	5:45
3:45	6:00
3:55	6:15
4:00	6:24
4:04	6:30
4:13	6:45
4:15	6:48
4:23	7:00
4:30	7:12
4:41	7:30
4:45	7:36
4:50	7:45
5:00	8:00
6:00	9:36
7:00	11:12

COMMONLY USED TERMS

The following terms are commonly used in running and podiatry circles. We provide short descriptions here and further explain them in the book, when necessary.

Achilles tendinosis: The chronic condition where there is thickening and scar tissue within the Achilles tendon if the Achilles tendonitis (below) is not properly rehabilitated.

Achilles tendon: The tendon that connects the calf muscles (gastrocnemius and soleus) to the heel bone. It is the thickest tendon in the human body.

Achilles tendonitis: An inflammation of the Achilles tendon.

Aponeurosis: A dense, fibrous connective tissue that attaches sheet-like muscles needing a wide area of attachment; for example, the plantar fascia.

Cadence: The number of landings per minute.

Calf muscles: The muscles that form the bulge on the back of the lower leg. These comprise the gastrocnemius (medial head and lateral head) and the flatter soleus underneath. These muscles are well developed in runners with good technique.

Chondromalacia patellae (runner's knee): A condition where the cartilage on the under-surface of the kneecap (patella) deteriorates and softens.

Cuboid: A cube-shaped bone on the lateral (outer) side of the foot, approximately half-way between the heel and the forefoot.

Dorsiflexion (of the foot): The foot position where the toes are stretched up towards the shin. This is opposite to plantarflexion.

Extensor tendons: The tendons on top of the foot.

Eversion (of the foot): The foot position where the sole arcs outwards.

Fibula: The thin bone that runs to the outside of the shin bone (tibia).

Gastrocnemius: see calf muscles.

Glutes (gluteus medius): One of three gluteal muscles in the buttocks, responsible for hip stability and countering internal rotation of the thigh. Glutes are well developed in runners with good technique.

Hamstrings: The long muscles at the back of the thigh.

Iliopsoas: Hip flexor muscle.

Iliotibial band (ITB): The fibrous sheath down the outside of the thigh, connecting the hip to the knee.

Inversion (of the foot): The foot position where the sole arcs inwards.

Medial longitudinal arch: Also known as the instep, this is the main arch of the foot.

Metatarsal heads: The foot 'knuckles', as seen in most feet when you curl your toes.

Metatarsophalangeal joint: The joint at the base of the toe and the metatarsal head.

Morton's neuroma: A painful condition producing nerve pain in the ball of the foot, most commonly between the third and fourth toes. It is due to thickened scar tissue in the sheath surrounding the nerve, which has become irritated and inflamed due to excess pressure, often simply from wearing narrow shoes.

Myofascia: Exceptionally strong, dense, flexible tissue that surrounds all muscles and bones.

Orthotics: An artificial support for the feet, to compensate for a biomechanical abnormality, and frequently used to prevent over-pronation. The long-term use of orthotics is associated with many skeletal injuries, and causes weakness in the feet.

Over-pronation: The situation where a runner's foot rolls too much inward when landing, and for an extended period of time. This is almost always due to over-striding.

Over-stride: The common situation where a runner's foot is making firm contact with the ground too far in front of the runner's hips. Reducing over-stride is the key to improving your running.

Peroneal muscles: The set of three muscles that both stabilise the lower leg and pronate the foot.

Plantar fascia: The thick fibrous band on the bottom of the foot, running from the heel to the five toes (see also *Illustration 60* in Appendix C).

Plantarflexion (of the foot): The foot position where the foot is stretched away from the shin (i.e. pointed). This is opposite to dorsiflexion.

Pronation: Refers to the foot rolling inward towards the inner edge of the sole. It is essential for shock absorption and adaption to uneven ground.

Quadriceps (quads): The four muscles that make up the front of the thigh.

Soleus: See calf muscles.

Stride length: The distance between landings, which increases with speed. A long stride length should be due to height off the ground and speed, not by stretching out along the ground; otherwise the runner will be over-striding.

Supination: This describes how the foot rolls outward to the outer edge of the sole, becoming a rigid lever for take-off.

Tibia: The main shin bone.

Tibialis anterior: The stabilising muscle at the front of the shin that attaches to the foot. It both dorsiflexes (foot pointing towards the shin) and inverts the foot (sole arcing inwards).

Tibialis posterior: The key stabilising muscle of the lower leg that attaches to the arch of the foot. It supports the medial arch of the foot (the instep) and assists with supination.

Vastus medialis obliquus (VMO): A pear-shaped muscle just above, and to the inside of, the knee. It is the main stabilising muscle of the thigh (quadriceps).

REFERENCES

Kirby KA. (1997), Foot and lower extremity biomechanics, In *A ten-year collection of Precision Intricast newsletters*, Payson, AZ, Precision Intricast Inc., pp. 267–268.

McPoil TG and Hunt G (1995), Evaluation and management of foot and ankle disorders: present problems and future directions, *Journal of Orthopaedic & Sports Physical Therapy*, 21(6):381–388.

Hunt CG (1988), Physical therapy of the foot and ankle, *Clinics in physical therapy*, volume 15.

Hunt CG and McPoil TG (editors) (1995), second edition, *Physical therapy of the foot and ankle*, Churchill Livingstone, New York.

National Government of South Africa (2006), South African National Guidelines on School Uniforms, *Staatskoerant* 173. (http://www.polity.org.za/article/south-african-schools-act-national-guidelines-on-school-uniforms-notice-173-of-2006-2006-03-20)

Root Ml, Orien WP and Weed JH (1977), *Normal and abnormal functions of the foot* (Volume 2). Clinical Biomechanics Corp, Los Angeles, CA. (https://books.google.com.au/books/about/Normal_and_Abnormal_Function_of_the_Foot.html?id=CI-KQgAACAAJ&redir_esc=y)

LIST OF ILLUSTRATIONS

Illustration 1: Heel (**left**), midfoot (**middle**), and forefoot (**right**) landing examples. All three landing examples are over-strides. In each case, the runner is leaning back as they land. This causes them to slow down. 2

Illustration 2: The stress points (**dark areas**) caused by a heel-strike over-stride. The initial impact (**left**) and then stress points (**right**) are a result of braking, balancing and supporting multiple times the body weight. 3

Illustration 3: The stress points (**dark areas**) caused by a forefoot-strike over-stride. The initial impact (**left**) and then stress points (**right**) are a result of braking, balancing and supporting multiple times the body weight. 4

Illustration 4: The difference between over-striding (**left**) and running with good form (**right**). 7

Illustration 5: Lower-body rotation (**bottom arrow**) and upper-body counter-rotation (**top arrow**) caused by over-striding. 9

Illustration 6: Location of symptoms of over-striding in the foot. **1**. Damaged toes, **2**. Metatarsal head stress fracture, **3**. Forefoot soreness (metatarsalgia and burning feet), **4**. Blisters, **5**. Plantar fasciitis, **6**. Achilles tendonitis or tendinosis. 16

Illustration 7: **Left**. Windlass Stress Test that podiatrists use to diagnose plantar fasciitis. It involves stressing the plantar fascia (**dark area**). **Right**. Most shoes put your foot in the Windlass Stress Test stressed position all the time, even when standing. They also open up and load the metatarsal joints, exposing them to injury. 18

Illustration 8: Location of symptoms of over-striding across the body (numbering continues from symptoms listed in Illustration 6). **7**. Posterior tibial tendonitis, **8**. Peroneal tendonitis, **9**. Posterior shin splints, **10**. Anterior shin splints, **11**. Runner's knee, **12**. Iliotibial band friction syndrome, **13**. Tight iliotibial band, **14**. Tight quads, **15** Muscle imbalance—strong quads and weak glutes, **16**. Hip flexor pain, **17**. Bursitis of the hip, **18**. Back or neck tension, **19**. Shoulder tension. 19

Illustration 9: This illustration, taken from a real picture of an over-striding runner, shows how runners try to stop knee pain so they can run without pain. This is a recipe for disaster. Knee supports merely allow runners to continue pounding their body until a more serious injury incapacitates them! We predict this runner will develop hip flexor pain, a lower-leg stress fracture or will need knee or hip surgery at a young age. 25

Illustration 10: Balanced landing. Hips above foot—landing vertically aligned. 29

Illustration 11: Start of the landing (i.e. before fully landing). In a balanced landing, your foot will touch lightly in front of your hips in a slightly supinated position. Do not try to land like this—it will happen naturally once you learn to land balanced. 31

Illustration 12: Completed landing. In a balanced landing, when completed, your foot will fully land when it is under your hips. Do not try to land like this—it will happen naturally once you learn to land balanced. 31

Illustration 13: Over-striding (**left**) means you are pushing against your direction of travel and increasing stress (**dark areas**) on certain parts of your body. The nearer you are to vertical (**right**) when landing, the less force there is on your body and the more evenly that force is distributed. 32

Illustration 14: High-impact over-stride (**left**) compared to a balanced, spring-loaded landing (**right**). 33

Illustration 15: Samples of bad (**top**) and good (**bottom**) footprints. A smooth footprint is a sign of efficient running (of not having to push forwards each step). Photo by Stuart Greaves. 34

Illustration 16: If you try to extend your stride length by advancing your foot it will be in front when you land. Notice the runner is barely getting off the ground. 35

Illustration 17: Trying to increase your stride length by lifting your knee is also advancing your foot and 'walking' forwards. 35

Illustration 18: When running with good technique, the whole body leaves the ground. Note that this illustration is based on a runner travelling at 20 kilometres per hour, which causes the heel to spring up closer to the hips than at lower speeds. 36

Illustration 19: To accelerate, take off in a more forwards direction. This requires a stronger take-off. If your acceleration is rapid, you will naturally increase your cadence to spread the load... 38

Illustration 20: Whole-foot Landing and Rebound exercise. Land whole-foot (**left**, **middle**) and bounce off (**right**) the whole foot. Don't be too stiff or too soft. Feel the spring!... 45

Illustration 21: Elasticity in Your Legs exercise. Slowing the tempo stresses the quads (**dark area**), in a similar way to over-striding. 47

Illustration 22: Standing tall as you leave the ground is the strongest position to be in, just like a weightlifter pushing upwards. There should be a straight line through your ground-contact point, your hips and your head when you take off, and also when you land. Note that in a good take-off the 'free' foot is also aligned with the grounded foot, the hips and the head. 50

Illustration 23: Bouncing and Tilting in Different Directions exercise. Bouncing on both feet (**left**) and then doing a whole-body tilt sideways (**middle left**), backwards (**middle right**), and forwards (**right**). 51

Illustration 24: Single-leg Start exercise. Start off by standing on one leg and bounce and tilt to accelerate. Your foot will follow and then drop under your hips. Make sure that you land your heel. 54

Illustration 25: Acceleration by Taking Off More Strongly exercise. Increasing your take-off power by trying to go up will result in a longer stride and more speed. 57

Illustration 26: Acceleration by Tilting More exercise. Increasing your forwards tilt (**white arrow**) will induce a stronger take-off, giving a longer stride and more speed. 58

Illustration 27: Accelerating, showing degree of tilt (**white**) and amount of ground pressure (**down-arrows**). **Left**. Running and speeding up, with whole-body tilt forwards for more speed. **Right**. Running and slowing down, with whole-body tilt backwards to reduce speed. 59

Illustration 28: Butt Kicks with Exaggerated Forwards Tilt exercise steps. **Left**. An upright stance. **Middle**. High-frequency butt kicks with your knees held back. **Right**. Balancing on your toes with very little forwards motion. 63

Illustration 29: Butt Kicks Into a Fast Run exercise. **Left**. An upright stance. **Middle left**. High-frequency butt kicks with your knees held back. **Middle right**. Butt kicks with your feet landing behind your hips. **Right**. Removing the butt kick by gradually reducing the kick as you increase speed to the point where your feet are landing firmly under your hips. 65

Illustration 30: Back-foot Check exercise. Look behind you to check that your back foot is moving the right way. If you have habitually been a heel-striker then this should get you balanced. 69

Illustration 31: The 360-degree Spin exercise. While running, make a seamless spin like a dancer or ice skater. 70

Illustration 32: Uphill running. Simply standing up and making sure your heel is moving towards your hamstrings is all that is needed as a cue for most people to start running uphill with good form. 75

Illustration 33: The Pendulum (moving) exercise. The three alignments during the pendulum exercise. Depicted are multiple sets of backwards tilt, forwards tilt, then upright. Begin with the most pronounced (**A**) tilt then reduce the tilt in each set (**B**) and (**C**). 80

Illustration 34: Stand Tall and Reset exercise, correction method 3 for when you start to fatigue. While running, stand tall and then aim your heel at your hamstrings (think 'back of the knee' as a good approximation). 83

Illustration 35: Water check. This photo, taken just before the landing is completed, shows how the foot enters and leaves the water with minimum disturbance. The water from the splashes is near-vertical in response to the landings, which are also near-vertical. Photo by Stuart Greaves. 86

Illustration 36: A hard high-density spiky ball—available at sports stores and physio suppliers. Make sure it is hard, spiky and about 10 centimetres in diameter. Photo by Stuart Greaves. 93

Illustration **37**: The Maestro—Conduct the Orchestra exercise. Positions 1 to 3.96

Illustration 38: Birdie on a Wire exercise. Positions 1 to 5. 98

Illustration 39: Foot Bridges exercise. Positions 1 and 2. 99

Illustration 40: Toe Wave exercise (standing toe curl). Positions 1 to 3. 101

Illustration 41: Marble Mover exercise. Positions 1 to 4. 102

Illustration 42: Front of Shin and Ankle Stretch exercise. **Position 1**. stretch out the front of your shin, the top of your ankle and your extensor tendons. 104

Illustration 43: Front of Shin and Ankle Stretch exercise. **Position 2**. to intensify the stretch, rotate your foot out 90 degrees. 104

Illustration 44: Quarter Knee Squat exercise. Positions 1 and 2. 106

Illustration 45: Transitional soreness you may get as your body gets used to different pressures. This soreness will most commonly occur in the calves (**1**), foot arches (**2**) and Achilles tendons (**3**). 114

Illustration 46: Straight Leg – Bent Leg Calf Raise exercise (double-leg version shown). Rise up onto the balls of your feet (**left**) and hold this position for 45 seconds. Slowly bend your knees (**right**) and hold for another 45 seconds. 117

Illustration 47: Plantar Fascia Stretch exercise. 119

Illustration 48:. Adjustable ankle weight used in the Fixing Runner's Knee and Medial Meniscus Pain exercise. Photo by Stuart Greaves 122

Illustration 49: Fixing Runner's Knee and Medial Meniscus Pain exercise. Positions 1 to 5..................123

Illustration 50: Features of a good shoe. The right shoe has a 5–10 mm thin (**a**) and (**b**) sole, which is flat and flexible and provides a little cushioning and protection from heat, cold and rough ground..................127

Illustration 51: Features of a bad shoe. **a**. An unnecessarily thick and soft sole at the rear of the shoe, **b**. An unnecessarily thick sole under the midfoot, **c**. Drop (slope from heel to toe), **d**. A flared heel, **e**. A stiff or angled heel counter, **f**. A turned-up toe box area..................129

Illustration 52: Sole thickness. Compared to running barefoot (**left figure**), thick soles (**right figure**) reduce your ability to react to changing ground conditions. Thick soles increase the chances of ankle sprains (**dark area**) and knee twists (**dark area**) and create instability and more stress up the body..................130

Illustration 53: Cushioning. Landing and take-off angles in a barefoot runner (**top**) and a runner wearing a soft-soled shoe (**bottom**) show how the shod runner needs to land leaning backwards (braking) and take-off more forwards, with more effort..................131

Illustration 54: The drop. **Top**. A barefoot runner. **Bottom**. If your shoe has a drop, it is impossible to land with your body vertically aligned (**middle figure**). The raised heel will force a change in technique, make you land your foot further in front of you or, at best, leave you with your knee pushed forwards and your hips dropping lower (**arrows**). This semi-squat position prevents you from getting a rebound and so requires you to push forwards into the next over-stride (**right figure**)..................132

Illustration 55: Stress on the plantar fascia (**dark area**). **Left**. Stress caused by the Windlass Stress Test for plantar fasciitis. **Right**. The same stress caused by a chunky shoe with a turned-up toe box..................134

Illustration 56: A shoe with holes in the forefoot area (**1**) and middle (**2**), and different density sole segments (**3**). If a shoe is thin enough there is no need to make it more flexible with slits or holes..................135

Illustration 57: Good running produces a good body shape. The characteristics whereby you can recognise a good runner: **1**. A tight butt, **2**. Strong, 'cut' hamstrings and calf muscles, **3**. Core strength. **4**. Light shoes..................143

Illustration 58: Adapted from a photo of a young female runner. Poor running in chunky shoes produces a poor body shape: weak glutes, strong quads and a significant curve in the lower back. The vertical line through the ground-contact point shows most of her body is behind her foot..................145

Illustration 59: **A**. Correct posture. Thin, flat, flexible shoes and an upright, strong body with postural muscles engaged. **B**. Incorrect posture. Raising the heel makes you push your knees back and your hips forwards. **C**. Incorrect posture. Raising the heel makes you bend your knees and your lower back. In neither B nor C the spine is vertical. 177

Illustration 60: Parts of the plantar fascia (aponeurosis). **1**. Lateral band, **2**. Medial band, **3**. Central band..192

LIST OF EXERCISES

EXERCISE 5.1: Experimenting with Foot Contact 44

EXERCISE 5.2: Whole-foot Landing and Rebound 44

EXERCISE 5.3: Elasticity in Your Legs 46

EXERCISE 6.1: Bouncing and Tilting in Different Directions 50

EXERCISE 6.2: Bouncing on Alternate Feet 51

EXERCISE 6.3: Bouncing on Alternate Feet and Tilting to Start Your Run 52

EXERCISE 6.4: Single-leg Start 53

EXERCISE 7.1: Accelerating by Taking Off More Strongly 56

EXERCISE 7.2: Accelerating by Tilting More 57

EXERCISE 7.3: Accelerating by Raising the Back Foot 59

EXERCISE 8.1: Butt Kicks with Exaggerated Forwards Tilt 62

EXERCISE 8.2: Butt Kicks Into a Fast Run 64

EXERCISE 9.1: Starting Off 68

EXERCISE 9.2: Back-foot Check 68

EXERCISE 9.3: The 360-degree Spin 69

EXERCISE 9.4: Warm-Up 70

EXERCISE 9.5: Your Run 71

EXERCISE 10.1: Preparation for the Pendulum (stationary) 78

EXERCISE 10.2: The Pendulum (moving) 78

EXERCISE 10.3: The Acceleration Ladder 81

EXERCISE 10.4: Back-foot Adjustment 81

EXERCISE 10.5: Stand Tall and Reset 82

EXERCISE 10.6: Downhill Sprints 87

EXERCISE 10.7: Accelerating by Increasing Your Over-stride 88

EXERCISE 10.8: Accelerating by Increasing Your Cadence 88

EXERCISE 10.9: Accelerating by Getting Airborne 89

EXERCISE 11.1: The Spiky Ball 94

EXERCISE 11.2: The Maestro—Conduct the Orchestra! 95

EXERCISE 11.3: Birdie on a Wire 97

EXERCISE 11.4: Foot Bridges 98

EXERCISE 11.5: Toe Wave 100

EXERCISE 11.6: Marble Mover 101

EXERCISE 11.7: Front of Shin and Ankle Stretch 103

EXERCISE 11.8: Quarter Knee Squat 105

EXERCISE 13.1: Straight Leg – Bent Leg Calf Raise 116

EXERCISE 13.2: Plantar Fascia Stretch 119

EXERCISE 13.3: Fixing Runner's Knee and Medial Meniscus Pain 121

INDEX

This subject index has **bold** page numbers for illustrations, and *italicised* page numbers for exercises.

360-degree Spin exercise, *69*, **70**
accelerating, 37–38, **38**, 55–60, **59**
   and decelerating, 59
   coaching instructions, 165
   exercises, *55*, **57**, *58*, *59*
   in sprinting, 38
   initial take-off, 37
   treadmill exercises, 87–90
   while running, 37
Accelerating by Getting Airborne exercise, 89–90
Accelerating by Increasing Your Cadence exercise, 88
Accelerating by Increasing Your Over-stride exercise, 88
Accelerating by Raising the Back Foot exercise, *59*
Accelerating by Taking Off More Strongly exercise, 55–56, **57**
Accelerating by Tilting More exercise, *57*, **58**
Acceleration Ladder exercise, *81*
Achilles tendon
   changes during Muscle Rebuilding stage, 109
   transitional soreness, 114

Achilles tendonitis and tendinosis, 10, 18–19, 115, 124
   podiatry information, 180
   rehabilitation exercises, *92–94*, *95–104*, 115–17, *116–17*, **117**
ankle problems
   Front of Shin and Ankle Stretch exercise, *103*
   rehabilitation, 123–24
ankle weight, 121, **122**
anterior shin splints, **19**, 21
arm swing, 9–10, **9**, 169
asymmetry in body shape, 142
athlete's foot, 149
'baby giraffe syndrome', 140, 142
back pain, **19**, 23–24, 178, 183–84
Back-foot Adjustment exercise, *81–82*
Back-foot Check exercise, *68*, **69**
back-foot lifters, 169
balance point, 61–65, *see also* vertically-aligned landing
   The Pendulum exercise, *77–80*

balanced landing. *See* landing
barefoot running
    and reducing ankle sprains, **130**
    comparison with shoes, **130–31**, **131**, **132**
    during coaching, 163, 168
    during Early Days stage, 109
    to refine your form, 86–87, 124
    transition changes to expect from, 108
Bateman, Keith
    biography, xvii–xx, 158
beach check, 33, **34**, 84–85
biomechanics
    and body shape, 148
    and shoes, 156
    Dr Root theory, 172
Birdie on a Wire exercise, *97*, **98**
    podiatry information, 194
Blackman, David, 112
blisters, **16**, 17, 149
body care, 149–50
body shape. *See* runner's body; posture
Bouncing and Tilting in Different Directions exercise, *50*, **51**
Bouncing on Alternate Feet and Tilting to Start Your Run exercise, *52*
Bouncing on Alternate Feet exercise, *51*
bursitis of the hip. See hip problems
Butt Kicks Into a Fast Run exercise, *63–65*, **65**

Butt Kicks with Exaggerated Forwards Tilt exercise, *61–62*, **63**
cadence
    and reducing over-stride, 152–53
    and refining your form, 83
    downhill, 76
    during your run, *71*, *72–73*
    finding, 153
    uphill, 74
    when accelerating, 38, 55, 60, *88*
calf muscles, 18
    changes during transition, 108
    changes to expect, 109
    strengthening, *94*
    transitional soreness, 114
calf tears, 115, 117–18
    rehabilitation exercise, *116–17*
case studies
    Complicated case of plantar fasciitis, bilateral medial meniscus pain and lower back pain, 183–84
    Functional orthotics prescribed for flat feet, 181–82
    Heidi's own injuries, 185–87
Castiglione, Angelo, 190
change management. *See* transition management
checking your form, *77–90*
    Acceleration Ladder exercise, *81*
    adjusting spring and take-off power, 83

Back-foot Adjustment exercise, *81–82*
barefoot running on a hard surface, 86–87
beach check, 84–85
Downhill Sprints exercise, *87*
dusty-track check, 84
making it wrong to make it right, 84
Stand Tall and Reset exercise, *82–83*, **83**
The Pendulum exercise, *77–80*, **80**
treadmill exercises, 87–90
water check, 85–86, **86**
chondromalacia patellae. *See* runner's knee
clawed-toe deformity, *97, 100*, 177
coaching instructions, 158–70
  dealing with problems, 167
  for Keith's Lessons, 163–66
  general tips, 170
  post-session guidance, 167
  preparation for technique change, 159
  private sessions, 169
  theory, 160
compartment syndrome, 21
cool-down after running, 72
cross-training, 140–41
decelerating, 59
del Monaco, Gaetano, 190
distance running, 38, 72–73
downhill running, *56, 73, 75–76, 87*, 151
Downhill Sprints exercise, *87*
drinking, 149

drop (of shoe), **129**, 131–33, **132**
'duck feet', 141–42
dusty-track check, 84
Elasticity in Your Legs exercise, *43, 46*, **47**
exercises list, 213–14
Experimenting with Foot Contact exercise, *43, 44*
'falling' forwards, 154–55
Fixing Runner's Knee and Medial Meniscus Pain exercise, *121–22*, **122**, **123**
flat feet, 141
  and orthotics, 136, 175
  podiatry case study, 181–82
Foot Bridges exercise, *98–99*, **99**
  podiatry information, 194
foot problems and injuries
  and orthotics, 136, 175, 181–82
  and over-pronation, 10–11
  arch soreness, 114
  asymmetry, 142
  athlete's foot, 149
  blisters, **16**, 17, 149
  burning, **16**, 17
  duck feet, 141–42
  flat feet, 136, 141, 175, 181–82
  forefoot soreness, 17
  from over-striding, 16–19
  itchy feet, 149
  metatarsal head stress fracture, **16**, 17
  metatarsalgia, **16**, 17
  plantar fasciitis, **16**, 18
  toe problems, **16**, *97, 98–99, 100*

Foot Program, 95–104
    podiatry information, 193–95
foot strengthening, 92–94, 95–104
    Birdie on a Wire exercise, *97, 98*
    Foot Bridges exercise, *98–99, 99*
    Front of Shin and Ankle Stretch exercise, *103,* **104**
    Marble Mover exercise, *101–2,* **102**
    podiatry information, 178–80
    Spiky Ball exercise, *92–94*
    The Maestro exercise, *95–96, 96*
    Toe Wave exercise, *100,* **101**
foot strike, 154, see also over-striding
forefoot pain, **16**, 17, 124, 144, 177
forefoot-strike over-stride, **2**, 4, 17, 154, *see also* over-striding
form, checking of. See checking your form
Front of Shin and Ankle Stretch exercise, *103,* **104**
    podiatry information, 195
glossary, 203–5
gluteal muscles (glutes), 8, **19**, *see also* muscle imbalance
    podiatry information, 179–80, 195–96
    strengthening, 93, *104–6,* **106**, 141
goal setting, 155
good form. See technique, good; vertically-aligned landing

hallux adbucto valgus deformity, 177
heel spurs, 10
heel-strike over-stride, **2**, 3–4, **3**, 15, 17, 21, **69**, *see also* over-striding
  and shoes, 133
  coaching information, 166, 167
Heidi's rehabilitation exercises, 113–24
    Achilles tendon injuries, 115–17
    ankle pain, 123–24
    case studies, 181–88
    forefoot pain, 124
    knee problems, 120–23, **122**, **123**
    plantar fasciitis, 118–19
    podiatry information, 178–80
    transitional soreness, 114–15, **114**
Heidi's Strengthening Program, 91–106
    case studies, 181–88
    foot strengthening, 92–94, 95–104
    gluteal muscle strengthening, 104–6
    history, 189–90
    podiatry information, 178–80, 191–96
    sources, 190–91
hills, 73–76
    downhill running, *56,* 73, 75–76, 151
    Downhill Sprints exercise, *87*
    uphill running, 73–74, **75**

hip problems
   bursitis, **19**, 23
   flexor pain, **19**, 23
   hip-drop, 11, 180
Hunt, Gary, 173
iliotibial band
   friction syndrome, **19**, 22, 181–82
   repetitive stress, 11–12
   tightness, **19**, 22
illustrations list, 207–12
injuries. *See under specific injury terms*
injuries from poor technique, 15–25, see also under foot problems and injuries; and specific injury terms
   Achilles tendonitis and tendinosis, 18–19
   and over-pronation, 10–11
   anterior shin splints, **19**, 21
   back pain, **19**, 23–24
   blisters, **16**, 17, 149
   forefoot pain, 17
   hip pain, **19**, 23
   hip-drop, 11
   how to deal with, 24–25, 111
   iliotibial band problems, 11–12, **19**, 22
   metatarsal head stress fracture, **16**, 17
   muscle imbalance, **19**, 21, 22
   neck pain, **19**, 23–24
   peroneal tendonitis, **19**, 20
   plantar fasciitis, **16**, 17, **18**
   posterior shin splints, **19**, 20
   posterior tibial tendonitis posterior, 19
   quadriceps tightness, **19**, 22
   repetitive stress, 11–12
   runner's knee, **19**, 21–22
   shoulder pain, **19**, 24
   stress fractures, 21
   tibial tendonitis, posterior, **19**
   toe damage, **16**
itchy feet, 149
Jones, Christopher, 191
Jones, Heidi
   biography, xx–xxiv, 171, 189–90
   injury case study, 185–87
Keith's Game Changer, 61–65
   coaching instructions, 165
Keith's Lessons
   1. landing, 43–47
   2. take-off, 49–54
   3. accelerating, 55–60
   4. Keith's Game Changer, 61–65
   5. going for a run, 67–76
   6. maintaining good form, 77–90
   coaching instructions, 158–70
   overview, 39–41
kilometres to miles conversion chart, 202
Kirby, Kevin, 173
knee problems, 11–12, **25**
   and orthotics, 136
   rehabilitation, 120–23, **122**, **123**
   runner's knee, **19**, 21–22
knee-lifters, 168–69
landing, 28–32, 43–47
   and over-striding, 161
   balanced, 12, 28–29, **29**, **31**, **32**, 63–65, *77–80*

Butt Kicks Into a Fast Run
  exercise, *63–65*, **65**
*Butt Kicks with Exaggerated
  Forwards Tilt* exercise, *61–
  62*, **63**
coaching instructions, 164
Elasticity in Your Legs
  exercise, *43, 46*, **47**
*Experimenting with Foot
  Contact* exercise, *43, 44*
foot action, 30–32
vertical alignment, 8–9, **29**,
  161–62
*Whole-foot Landing and
  Rebound* exercise, *43, 44–
  46*, **45**
leg asymmetry, 142
leg injuries, 10–11, *see also
  under* injuries from poor
  technique
leg length, 13
lessons. *See* Keith's Lessons
lift-and-place runners, 168–69
lunges, 141
Maestro. *See* The Maestro
  exercise
Marble Mover exercise, *101–2*,
  102
  podiatry information, 195
McCloskey, Alan, 191
McPoil, Thomas, 173
medial meniscus pain, 120–23,
  122, 123, 136, 183–84, 187
medial tibial stress syndrome.
  See posterior shin splints
medical information. *See*
  podiatry information
meniscus pain, 120–23, ***122,
  123***, 136, 183–84, 187

metatarsal head stress fracture,
  16, 17
metatarsalgia, **16**, 17, 133, 177
midfoot-strike over-stride, **2**, 5,
  154
miles to kilometres conversion
  chart, 202
muscle imbalance, **19**, 21, 22,
  133, **145**
  and duck feet, 141
  and poor posture, 8, 144
myofascia, 192, 193
neck pain and tension, **19**, 23–
  24, 178
*Normal and abnormal functions
  of the foot*, 173, 175
orthotics, 136–37
  and over-pronation, 136
  and over-supination, 136,
    183, 187
  and plantar fasciitis, 187–88
  and podiatry, 172–73, 173–
    75, 175–76
  and shoes, 162–63
over-pronation
  and orthotics, 136
  and over-striding, 11
  and shoes, 134, 156
  injuries caused by, 10–11, 20
over-striding, 1, **2, 7, 32**, *see also*
  technique, poor
  *Accelerating by Increasing Your
    Over-stride* exercise, 88
  and downhill running, 75–76
  and knee supports, **25**
  and stride length, 152
  and upper-body rotation, 9–
    10
  coaching instructions, 161

defined, 2–5
forefoot-strike, **2**, 4, 15, 17, 154
heel-strike, **2**, 3–4, **3**, 15, 17, 21, **69**, 133, 166, 167
high impact take-off, **33**
how to check, 5–6
injuries caused by, 15–25
midfoot-strike, **2**, 5, 154
upper-body rotation, **9**
OYF Rules, 197–201
Rule 1, Get a side-view video regularly, 5–6
Rule 2, Stand and land aligned, 8
Rule 3, Over-pronation is a symptom of over-striding, 11
Rule 4, Bounce and fly, 12
Rule 5, Spring, don't swing, 13
Rule 6, Fix the problem not the symptom, 24
Rule 7, Hips first—your foot will follow, 34
Rule 8, Don't try to control your feet, 36, 37
Rule 9, Aim for balanced whole-foot landings, 45–46
Rule 10, Drills and exercises should directly relate to running actions, 140–41
OYF Running, xxv, xxvi, 27–38
coaching instructions, 158–70
peroneal tendonitis, 10, **19**, 20, 123, 124
plantar fascia, **18**, 192–93, **192**

Plantar Fascia Stretch exercises, *118*, *119*
plantar fasciitis, 10, **16**, 17, **18**
and orthotics, 187–88
rehabilitation exercises, *92–94*, *95–104*, *118–19*, *119*
podiatry information, 171–88
'accepted wisdom', 172–73
for Heidi's Strengthening Program, 189–96
questioning 'accepted wisdom', 173–75, 175–76
treating runners, 176–78
posterior shin splints, **19**, 20, 21
posterior tibial tendon, 19, 20, 109, 123, 182
posterior tibial tendonitis, 10, **19**, 123, 180
posture
change during transition, 108
correct vs incorrect, 176–78, **177**
good form, 142, **143**
poor form, 8–9, 144, **145**
pronation, 10, 30, *see also* over-pronation
quadriceps muscles (quads), 8, *see also* muscle imbalance
and elasticity, *46*, **47**
tightness, **19**, 22
Quarter Knee Squat exercise, *104–5*, **106**, 141
podiatry information, 179–80, 195–96
race walking, 12
racing, 150–51
rehabilitation. *See* Heidi's rehabilitation exercises

repetitive stress, 11–12
Root, Merton, 172
runner's knee (chondromalacia patellae), **19**, 21–22, 120
   rehabilitation exercise, 121–22
runner's body, how to get, 139–45
   body strength, 140
   good form, 142–44
   training, 140–42
running injuries. See injuries from poor technique
running lesson, 67–76, *see also* running tips
   360-degree Spin exercise, *69, 70*
   Back-foot Check exercise, *68, 69*
   building distance, 72–73
   checking your form, 68–70, 77–90
   coaching instructions, 166
   cool-down, 72
   hills, 73–76
   stages of a run, 70–73
   Starting Off exercise, *68*
   Warm-Up exercise, *70*
   Your Run exercise, *71–72*
running technique. See technique, poor; technique, good
running tips, 147–57
Sever's disease, 19
shin splints. See posterior shin splints; anterior shin splints

shoes, 125–37
   and biomechanics, 156
   and orthotics, 136–37, 162–63, see also under orthotics
   and poor technique, 7–8
   bad features, 128–29, **129–35**
   cushioning, 130–31
   drop, **129**, 130, 131–33, **132**
   during transition, 112
   good features, 127–28
   heel counter, 133
   heel flare, 133
   influence on body shape, 176–78, **177**
   injuries from bad shoes, 17, 18, 21, 23, 129–35
   sole density, splits and holes, 135
   sole stiffness, 134
   sole thickness, 130
   technological features in, 126
   testing, 156
   toe box, 133–34, 134–35
   weight, 135
shoulder swing, 9–10, **9**, 169
shoulder tension, **19**, 24
Single-leg Start exercise, *52–53, 54*
spiky ball, **93**, *92–94*
Spiky Ball exercise, *94*
   podiatry information, 192–93
spring in legs
   adjusting, 83
   Elasticity in Your Legs exercise, *43, 44,* **47**
   in take-off, **33**

in whole-foot, vertically-
aligned landing, 45, 162
sprinters, 38
stair running, 141
Stand Tall and Reset exercise,
 82–83, **83**
Starting Off exercise, *68*
Straight Leg – Bent Leg Calf Raise
 exercise, *116–17*, **117**
strengthening. See Heidi's
 Strengthening Program
stress fractures, 10, **16**, 17, 21
stride length, **35**, **36**, 55–60, 60,
 152, 161
  calculation, 152
supination, 10, 20, 30
take-off, 32–37, 49–54
  and landing, 36
  and spring, **33**, 83
  and standing tall, **50**
  Bouncing and Tilting in
   Different Directions
   exercise, *50*, **51**
  *Bouncing on Alternate Feet
   and Tilting to Start Your Run*
   exercise, *52*
  Bouncing on Alternate Feet
   exercise, *51*
  coaching instructions, 164–
   65
  Single-leg Start exercise, *52–
   53*, **54**
technique. See technique, poor;
 technique, good
technique change, xxv–xxvi,
 107–12, *see also* Keith's
 Lessons
  changes to expect, 107–8
  coaching instructions, 158–
   70
  Early Days stage, 108–9
  main points of, 110–12
  maintaining good form, 77–
   90, 166
  Muscle Rebuilding stage,
   109–10
  personal story, 112
  Reaping the Benefits stage,
   110
  strengthening during, 91–
   106
  tips and traps, 147–57
technique, good, 27–38, *see also*
 Keith's Lessons
  accelerating, 37–38
  body strength, 140
  landing, 28–32
  maintaining, 77–90
  posture, 142–44, **143**
  take-off, 32–37
  vs poor technique, 87–90
technique, poor, 1–13
  and shoes, 7–8
  how to check, 5–6
  injuries caused by, 15–25
  over-striding, 2–5
  posture, 144, **145**
  run don't walk, 12–13
  signs of, 6–12
  vs good technique, 87–90
The Maestro exercise, *95–96*, **96**
  podiatry information, 193–94
The Pendulum exercise, *77–80*,
 80
tibialis anterior muscle, 21, 100,
 103, 194

tibialis posterior muscle, 20, *101*
tibialis posterior tendon. *See* posterior tibial tendon
tips. *See* running tips
toe problems, **16**
   clawed-toe deformity, *97, 100*
   rehabilitation exercises, *97, 98–99, 100*
Toe Wave exercise, *100,* **101**
   podiatry information, 194
toe-runners, 168
trail running, 151
training, 147–48, *see also* running lesson
   during transition, 111
   things not to worry about, 140–42
transition management, 107–12
   changes to expect, 107–8
   Early Days stage, 108–9
   main points, 110–12
   Muscle Rebuilding stage, 109–10
   Reaping the Benefits stage, 110
   soreness, 114–15, **114**
treadmill exercises, 87–90
   Accelerating by Getting Airborne, 89–90

Accelerating by Increasing Your Cadence exercise, 88
Accelerating by Increasing Your Over-stride exercise, 88
tripping, 11
uphill running, 73–74, **75**
upper-body rotation, 9–10, **9**
vastus medialis obliquus, 120
vertical oscillation, 154
vertically-aligned landing, 8–9, **29**, *see also* landing
   and over-striding, **32**
   and shoe drop, 132
   and side-view video, 5–6
   coaching instructions, 161–62
   finding the balance point, 63–65, 77–80
video, side-view, 5–6, 151
   during transition, 111
   landing, 28–29
vitamins, 149
walking versus running, 12–13
warm-up, 70–71
   Warm-Up exercise, *70*
water check, 85–86, **86**
Whole-foot Landing and Rebound exercise, *43, 44–46,* **45**
Windlass Stress Test, **18**, 134
Your Run exercise, *71–72*

Printed in Great Britain
by Amazon